anatomy of
EXERCISE
FOR WOMEN

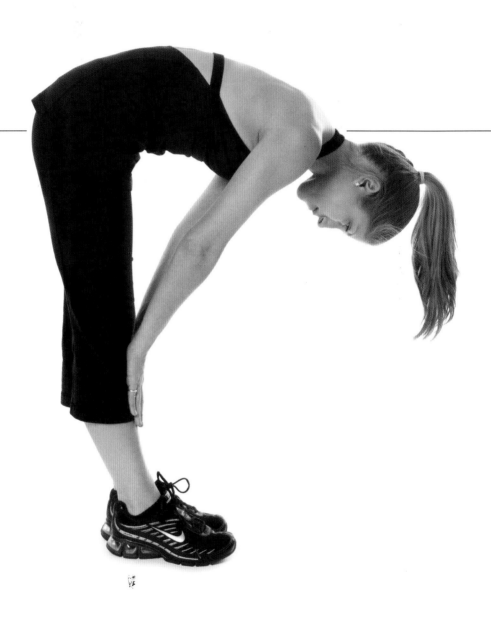

anatomy of
EXERCISE
FOR WOMEN

Lisa Purcell

hinkler

Note
Whilst every effort has been made to ensure that the content of this book is as technically accurate and as sound as possible, neither the author nor the publishers can accept responsibility for any injury or loss sustained as a result of the use of this material.

Published by Hinkler Books Pty Ltd 2014
45–55 Fairchild Street
Heatherton Victoria 3202 Australia
www.hinkler.com.au

hinkler

This book is produced using paper that is made from wood grown in managed, sustainable forests. It is natural, renewable and recyclable. The logging and manufacturing processes conform to the environmental regulations of the country of origin.

Printed and bound in China.

CONTENTS

Introduction: Fit & Feminine 9

Full-Body Anatomy 12

FLEXIBILITY EXERCISES 15

Neck Side Bend 16

Triceps Stretch 17

Posterior Hand Clasp 18

Chest Stretch 20

Swiss Ball Kneeling Lat Stretch 21

Latissimus Dorsi Stretch 22

Toe Touch 24

Cat and Dog Stretch. 26

Piriformis Stretch 28

Hip Stretch 29

Hip-to-Thigh Stretch 30

Spine Stretch 31

Swiss Ball Hip Crossover 32

Knee-to-Chest Hug. 34

Iliotibial Band Stretch. 36

Quadriceps Stretch 37

Standing Hamstrings Stretch 38

Standing Calf Stretch 39

Child's Pose 40

UPPER-BODY EXERCISES 43

Chair Dip 44

Chair Crunch 46

Overhead Press. 48

Alternating Chest Press 50

Standing Fly 52

Upwards Plank 54

Swiss Ball Pullover 56

Swiss Ball Triceps Extension 58

Swiss Ball Fly 60

Push-Up 62

Prone Trunk Raise 64

Dumbbell Upright Row 66

Alternating Dumbbell Curl 68

CORE-TRAINING EXERCISES 71

Crunch 72

Half Curl 74

Seated Russian Twist 76

Spine Twist 78

Oblique Roll-Down 80

Bicycle Crunch 82

The Boat 84

V-Up 86

Backwards Ball Stretch 88

Plank 90

Swiss Ball Transverse Abs 92

Swiss Ball Rollout 94

Foam Roller Calf Press 96

Foam Roller Diagonal Crunch 98

Foam Roller Supine Marches 100

Tiny Steps 102

Double-Leg Abdominal Press 104

The Twist 106

Standing Knee Crunch 108

Power Squat 110

CONTENTS continued

Swiss Ball Reverse Bridge Rotation 112

Swiss Ball Sitting Balance 114

Swiss Ball Hip Circles 116

Swiss Ball Reverse Bridge Roll 118

Abdominal Hip Lift 120

Leg Raise 122

LOWER-BODY EXERCISES 125

Foam Roller Iliotibial Band Release 126

Swiss Ball Jackknife 128

Shoulder Bridge 130

Foam Roller Bicycle 132

Single-Leg Circles 134

Scissors. 136

Wall Sits 138

Stiff-Legged Deadlift. 140

Forwards Lunge 142

Lateral Lunge 144

Dumbbell Lunge. 146

Dumbbell Calf Raise 148

Kneeling Side Lift 150

Put It All Together: Workouts. 153

Glossary. 158

Credits & Acknowledgements 160

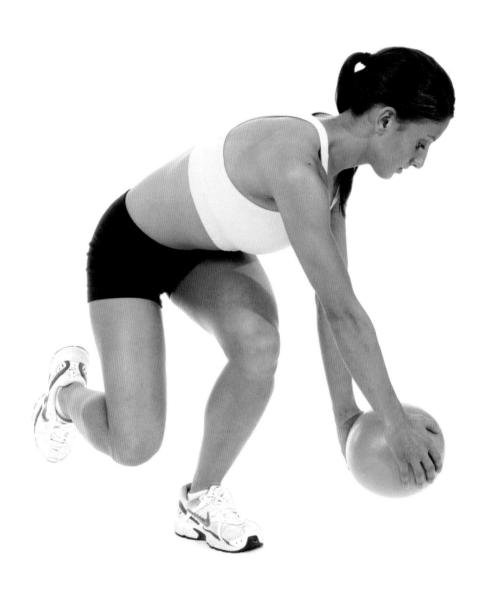

INTRODUCTION: FIT & FEMININE

Ever-increasing numbers of women are taking up fitness programmes, whether joining gyms,

running in marathons, or simply spreading a mat in the living room and trying out some

home exercise. The reasons are many: some women want to drop a few pounds and tone up

their thighs to fit into those skinny jeans; others are looking to improve their overall health

and increase their energy levels; some use exercise to manage stress and improve their

mood; and of course, many begin working out for a combination of all those reasons. The

simple fact is exercise makes us all feel better – and look better, too.

For whatever reason you've decided to follow an exercise programme, you'll find plenty of

valuable information and tips in the following pages. You'll find a guide to a comprehensive

exercise programme, devised with attention to your whole-body anatomy. The first group of

exercises focuses on flexibility, demonstrating moves that can warm you up before a longer

workout or just get you going to start your day. Sections on the upper body, the core and

the lower body target those areas most of us want to improve. Performed together, these

exercises will not only enhance your figure, but also increase you body's performance levels.

FIT & FEMININE

Fit and feminine: the goal for most women undertaking an exercise programme. We all want to look our best and feel our best, too, so that we can perform at peak levels, with energy to spare. With women's busy lives, it isn't always easy to fit in everything that needs to be done in a day, but making time to exercise is one of the best investments you can make in yourself.

MAKE TIME FOR FITNESS

All too often we put off starting an exercise programme because there simply doesn't seem to be enough time in a day. Yet, it may be easier than you think. For example, using this book as a guide, you can work out at home, saving the extra time (and money) that working out at a gym demands. Just find yourself a space (the living room, for instance), and set aside just 10 to 30 minutes a day, two or three times a week. Designate a regular time (say, after dinner); this encourages you to stick to a consistent schedule. Just as you can build up the weight on your dumbbells, so too can you build up the hours per week you spend exercising. Dip into this book over time, and don't be afraid to try something new; you may find an exercise that challenges you in a new way or discover that you're weak or strong in an area you never knew existed. Pay attention to what your limits are, and then work toward exceeding them. As you get more comfortable with the workout, devote more time to it to see faster, better results.

GETTING STARTED

Although you may be tempted to dive right into your workout, warming up is essential to any exercise programme. Warm-ups will increase the benefits of exercising and help decrease the potential of sustaining injury. The basic kinds of warm-ups fall into two categories: cardiovascular exercises and stretches. Cardio exercises stimulate blood and oxygen flow through your body. Try running in place, skipping, spinning or cycling, or even brisk

WORKING IN NEUTRAL

Neutral spine, also known as neutral posture, is an important concept that you need to understand before you begin practising exercising. Neutral spine is crucial for ensuring that you properly target and strengthen the muscles of the core, and it also keeps you in a more efficient position for movement.

Neutral spine is the proper alignment of the body between postural extremes. In its natural alignment, the spine is not straight. It has curves in the cervical (neck), thoracic (upper) and lumbar (lower) regions. Neutral alignment helps to cushion the spine from too much stress and strain. Controlling pelvic tilt is one way to begin helping to balance the spine. As certain muscles of the back and abdomen contract, the pelvis rotates. As the pelvis rotates backward, the lumbar curve increases. As the pelvis rotates forward, the curve of the low back straightens.

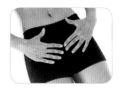

To find neutral spine while lying on your back, place your thumbs on your hip bones and your fingers over the pubic bone (the bone between your legs), creating a triangle. All the bones should line up on the same plane—no tipping back or to one side should be present. The triangle should appear flat, with all corners on the same plane. This position will prepare you for exercising when you are lying on your back.

If you are exercising on your stomach, you can find the neutral spine by pressing your pubic bone into the floor until you feel your back flatten slightly or your stomach lightly lift off the floor. Tuck your chin so that your forehead has contact with the surface, and your neck is now ready for strengthening. This position not only protects your back and your neck as you exercise, but it also allows you to exercise more productively. Maintaining neutral posture will help decrease the risk of injury and increase the efficiency of movement or exercise.

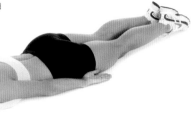

EXERCISE EXTRAS

To add variety to your fitness regimen, take advantage of everyday objects around the house: use a chair as a prop for dips and crunches, for instance, or take advantage of steps for lunges and calf exercises.

Many of the featured exercises incorporate equipment—all reasonably small tools that add variety and challenge to your workout.

Hand weights and dumbbells. Several of the toning exercises call for small hand weights or dumbbells. You can start with very light, 1-kilogram 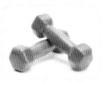 weights (or even lighter substitutes, such as unopened food cans or water bottles), and then work your way up to heavier ones. Both hand weights and dumbbells add resistance, increasing the benefits of many exercises. You can use either one for any exercise that calls for a weight. If you decide to invest in a set of dumbbells, look for an adjustable model that allows you to easily vary the weight levels.

Be sure it comes with a solid-locking mechanism that makes adding and subtracting weight discs fast and easy.

Medicine ball. A small, weighted medicine ball, which is used like a free weight, can also be used in any exercise that calls for a hand weight.

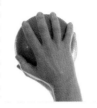

Swiss ball. Also known as an exercise ball, fitness ball, body ball, or balance ball, this heavy-duty inflatable ball is available in a variety of sizes, with diametres ranging from 30 to 75 centimetres. Be sure to find the best size for your height and weight. A Swiss ball is an excellent fitness aid that really works your core. Because it is unstable, you must constantly adjust your balance while performing a movement, which helps you improve your overall sense of balance and your flexibility.

Resistance band. Also known as "fitness band", "Thera-Band", "Dyna-Band", "stretching band" and "exercise band," this simple tool adds resistance to an exercise. You will see two types of resistance bands, one with handles and one without; both are amazing pieces of fitness equipment, which effectively tone and strengthen your entire body. Bands act in a similar way to hand weights, but unlike weights, which rely on gravity to determine the resistance, bands use constant tension—supplied by your muscles—to add resistance to your movements and improve your overall coordination.

Foam roller. Rollers come in a variety of sizes, materials and densities, and they can be used for stretching, strengthening, balance training, stability training and self-massage. If you do not have access to a foam roller, you can substitute a swimming noodle or a homemade towel roller. To make a towel roller, place two bath towels together, firmly roll them lengthwise, and then wrap the ends with tape. Although a towel roller works well, the dense foam of the roller will provide you with the best results.

walking. Stretches, such as those found in the first chapter, gradually and smoothly lengthen the muscles, maximising their flexibility.

HOW TO USE THIS BOOK

In the step-by-step chapters of this book, you'll find photos with instructions demonstrating how to execute each exercise and some tips on what to do to perform it correctly—and what to avoid. Some exercises have accompanying variations, shown in the modification box. Alongside each exercise is a quick-read panel that lists the exercise's major target, level of difficulty, and benefits. Also included is a list of precautions: if you have one of the issues listed, it is best to avoid that exercise. Each exercise also features illustrations showing key muscles. As you work out, visualise the muscles that you are engaging—it will help you maintain optimal form.

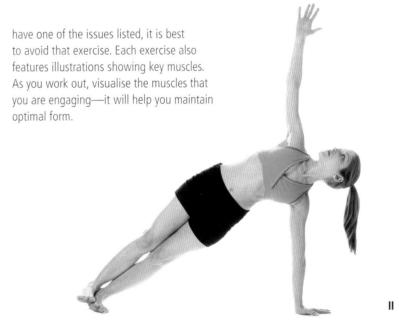

FULL-BODY ANATOMY

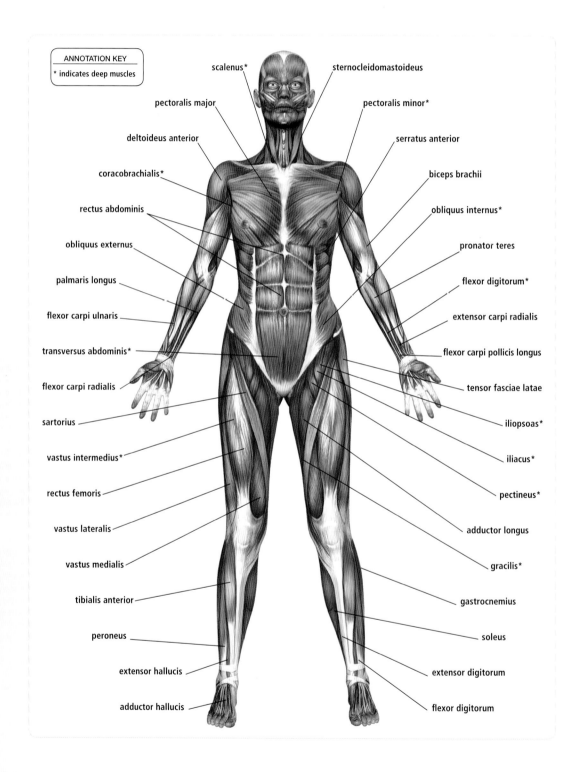

ANNOTATION KEY
* indicates deep muscles

scalenus*

sternocleidomastoideus

pectoralis major

pectoralis minor*

deltoideus anterior

serratus anterior

coracobrachialis*

biceps brachii

rectus abdominis

obliquus internus*

obliquus externus

pronator teres

palmaris longus

flexor digitorum*

flexor carpi ulnaris

extensor carpi radialis

transversus abdominis*

flexor carpi pollicis longus

flexor carpi radialis

tensor fasciae latae

sartorius

iliopsoas*

vastus intermedius*

iliacus*

rectus femoris

pectineus*

vastus lateralis

adductor longus

vastus medialis

gracilis*

tibialis anterior

gastrocnemius

peroneus

soleus

extensor hallucis

extensor digitorum

adductor hallucis

flexor digitorum

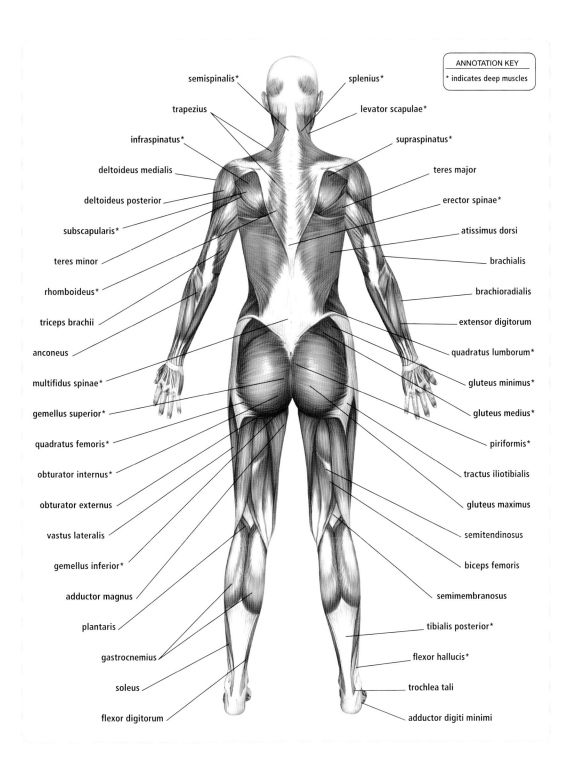

semispinalis*

splenius*

trapezius

levator scapulae*

infraspinatus*

supraspinatus*

deltoideus medialis

teres major

deltoideus posterior

erector spinae*

subscapularis*

atissimus dorsi

teres minor

brachialis

rhomboideus*

brachioradialis

triceps brachii

extensor digitorum

anconeus

quadratus lumborum*

multifidus spinae*

gluteus minimus*

gemellus superior*

gluteus medius*

quadratus femoris*

piriformis*

obturator internus*

tractus iliotibialis

obturator externus

gluteus maximus

vastus lateralis

semitendinosus

gemellus inferior*

biceps femoris

adductor magnus

semimembranosus

plantaris

tibialis posterior*

gastrocnemius

flexor hallucis*

soleus

trochlea tali

flexor digitorum

adductor digiti minimi

ANNOTATION KEY

* indicates deep muscles

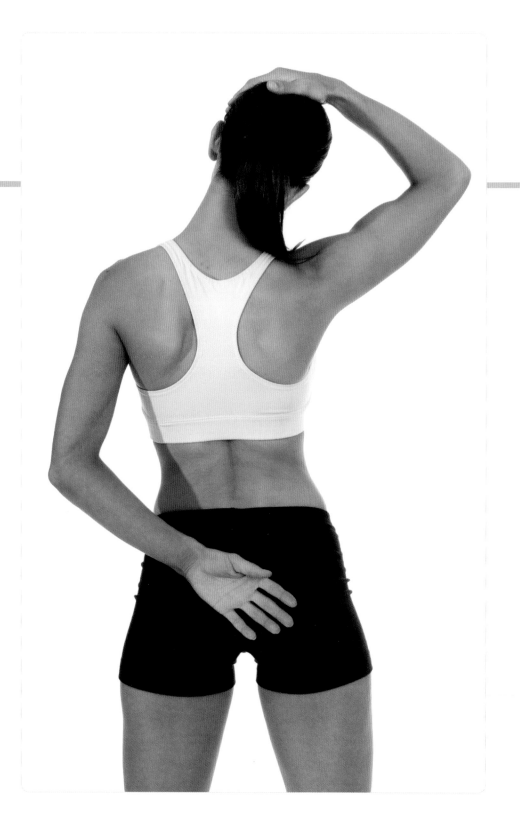

FLEXIBILITY EXERCISES

Flexibility improves your performance when you bend, lift and reach your way through daily life. Becoming more flexible can improve your physical performance and decrease your risk of injury. And, yes, we are all born with natural flexibility in certain areas but face challenges in others, but flexibility can always be improved over time and with practice. The following exercises all deliver targeted stretches to key muscles, and performing several before a workout is a great way to warm up. But stretching isn't just about warming up—regular stretching imparts multiple benefits. It can help relieve stress, for example, as well as combat the effects of ageing, improve muscle coordination, relieve lower-back pain and elongate muscles, making you look sleeker and fitter.

NECK SIDE BEND

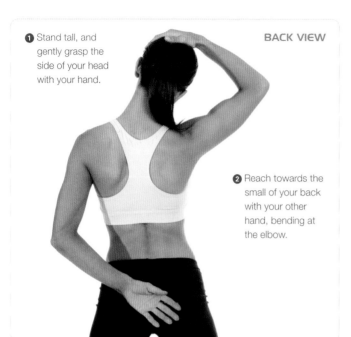

❶ Stand tall, and gently grasp the side of your head with your hand.

BACK VIEW

❷ Reach towards the small of your back with your other hand, bending at the elbow.

ANNOTATION KEY

Black text indicates target muscles

Grey text indicates other working muscles

* indicates deep muscles

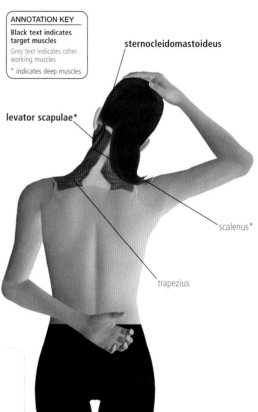

sternocleidomastoideus

levator scapulae*

scalenus*

trapezius

TARGETS
• Neck muscles

LEVEL
• Beginner

BENEFITS
• Increases neck flexibility

NOT ADVISABLE IF YOU HAVE . . .
• Severe neck pain

FRONT VIEW

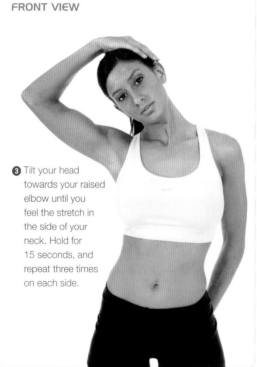

❸ Tilt your head towards your raised elbow until you feel the stretch in the side of your neck. Hold for 15 seconds, and repeat three times on each side.

AVOID
• Tensing or lifting your shoulders.
• Using your hand to tug your head downwards.

DO IT RIGHT
• Breathe easily and normally throughout the stretch.

BEST FOR

• levator scapulae
• sternocleidomastoideus

TRICEPS STRETCH

1 Stand tall keeping your neck, torso and shoulders straight.

2 Raise your right arm, and bend it behind your head.

3 Keeping your shoulders relaxed, grasp your raised elbow with your left hand, and gently pull back.

4 Continue to pull your elbow back until you feel the stretch on the underside of your arm. Hold for 15 seconds.

5 Repeat three times on each arm.

BACK VIEW

FRONT VIEW

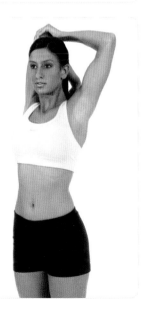

BEST FOR

- triceps brachii
- infraspinatus
- teres major
- teres minor

DO IT RIGHT
- Keep your dropped elbow close to the side of your head.

AVOID
- Leaning backwards.

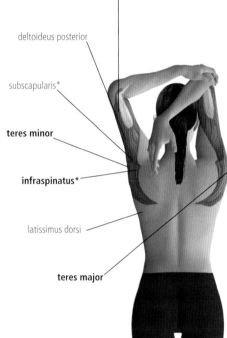

triceps brachii

deltoideus posterior

subscapularis*

teres minor

infraspinatus*

latissimus dorsi

teres major

TARGETS
- Shoulders
- Triceps

LEVEL
- Beginner

BENEFITS
- Improves range of motion

NOT ADVISABLE IF YOU HAVE . . .
- Shoulder instability

ANNOTATION KEY

Black text indicates target muscles

Grey text indicates other working muscles

* indicates deep muscles

POSTERIOR HAND CLASP

❶ Stand tall, keeping your neck, shoulders and torso straight. Your arms should hang loosely at your sides.

❷ Extend your right hand to the side, parallel to the floor.

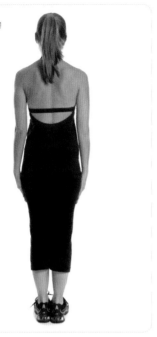

TARGETS
- Upper back
- Upper arms

LEVEL
- Intermediate

BENEFITS
- Stretches the shoulders, chest and upper arms

NOT ADVISABLE IF YOU HAVE . . .
- Shoulder injury

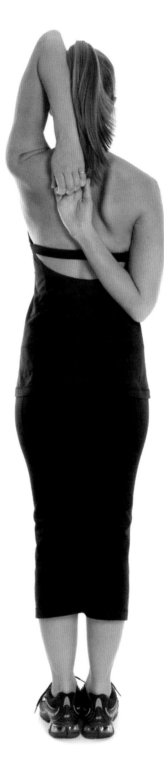

❸ Bend your elbow, and rotate your shoulder downward so that the palm of your hand faces outwards. Reach behind your back, palm still up, and draw your elbow into your right side.

❹ Continue to rotate your shoulder downward as you reach upwards with your hand until your forearm is parallel to your spine. Your right hand should rest in between your shoulder blades.

❺ Reach your left arm up with your palm facing directly behind you. Bend your elbow, reaching your left hand down the centre of your back.

❻ Hook your hands together behind your back. Lift your chest, and pull your abdominals in towards your spine.

❼ Hold for about 30 seconds to 1 minute. Release your arms, and repeat with your arms reversed for the same length of time.

AVOID
- Straining—if you cannot hook your hands behind your back, try using a strap or an elastic exercise band to help you pull your hands closer together.

DO IT RIGHT
- Keep your lower elbow tucked close to the side of your torso.

BEST FOR

- rhomboideus
- teres minor
- subscapularis
- latissimus dorsi
- deltoideus anterior
- deltoideus medialis
- deltoideus posterior
- triceps brachii
- pectoralis major
- pectoralis minor

ANNOTATION KEY

Black text indicates target muscles

Grey text indicates other working muscles

* indicates deep muscles

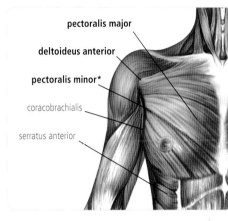

pectoralis major

deltoideus anterior

pectoralis minor*

coracobrachialis

serratus anterior

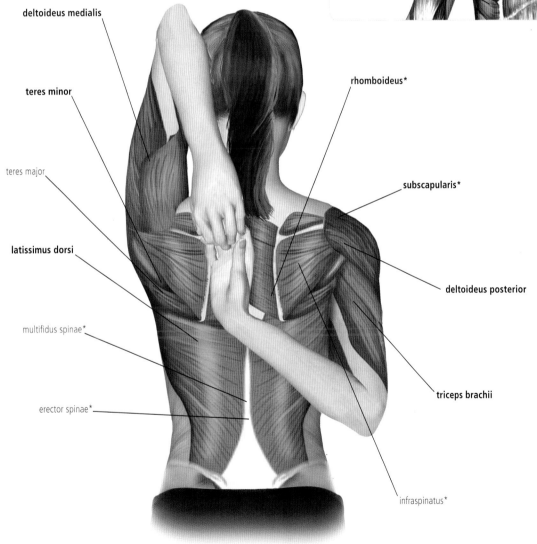

deltoideus medialis

teres minor

teres major

latissimus dorsi

multifidus spinae*

erector spinae*

rhomboideus*

subscapularis*

deltoideus posterior

triceps brachii

infraspinatus*

CHEST STRETCH

❶ Stand with your hands behind your head, with fingers interlocked. Your elbows should be pointing outwards.

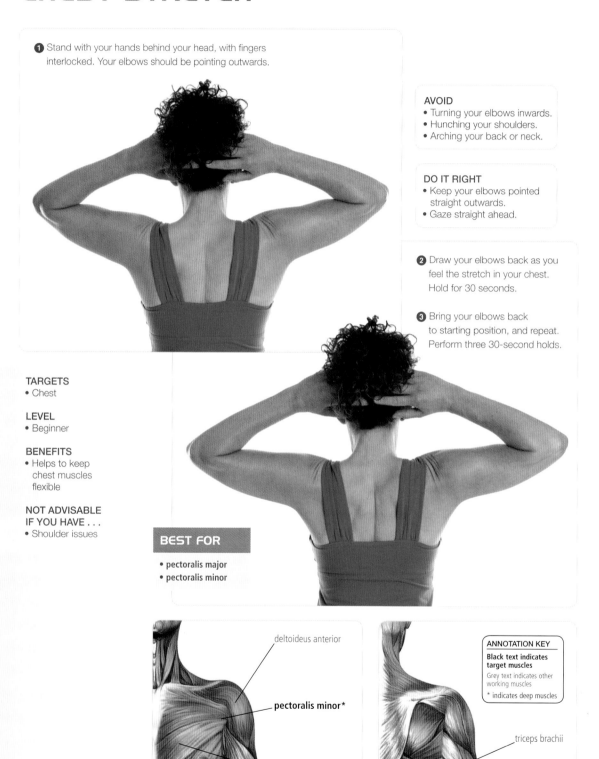

AVOID
- Turning your elbows inwards.
- Hunching your shoulders.
- Arching your back or neck.

DO IT RIGHT
- Keep your elbows pointed straight outwards.
- Gaze straight ahead.

❷ Draw your elbows back as you feel the stretch in your chest. Hold for 30 seconds.

❸ Bring your elbows back to starting position, and repeat. Perform three 30-second holds.

TARGETS
- Chest

LEVEL
- Beginner

BENEFITS
- Helps to keep chest muscles flexible

NOT ADVISABLE IF YOU HAVE . . .
- Shoulder issues

BEST FOR
- pectoralis major
- pectoralis minor

deltoideus anterior

pectoralis minor*

pectoralis major

triceps brachii

ANNOTATION KEY
Black text indicates target muscles
Grey text indicates other working muscles
* indicates deep muscles

SWISS BALL KNEELING LAT STRETCH

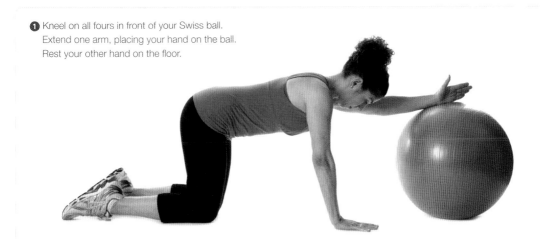

1 Kneel on all fours in front of your Swiss ball. Extend one arm, placing your hand on the ball. Rest your other hand on the floor.

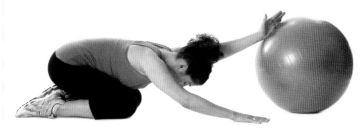

2 Lean back onto your heels until you feel a deep stretch in large muscles on either side of your back. Hold for 30 seconds.

3 Switch arms, and repeat. Complete three 30-second holds per arm.

BEST FOR

- latissimus dorsi
- erector spinae

TARGETS
- Back

LEVEL
- Beginner

BENEFITS
- Helps to keep back muscles flexible

AVOID IF YOU HAVE . . .
- Lower-back issues

AVOID
- Allowing your torso to twist.
- Arching your neck.

DO IT RIGHT
- Keep your arm fully extended on the ball.
- Face the floor throughout the stretch.

infraspinatus*

supraspinatus*

deltoideus posterior

teres minor

subscapularis*

triceps brachii

latissimus dorsi

erector spinae*

ANNOTATION KEY
Black text indicates target muscles
Grey text indicates other working muscles
* indicates deep muscles

LATISSIMUS DORSI STRETCH

1 Stand, keeping your neck, shoulders and torso straight.

2 Raise both arms above your head and clasp your hands together, palms facing upwards.

AVOID
- Leaning backwards as you come to the top of the circle.

DO IT RIGHT
- Elongate your arms and shoulders as much as possible.

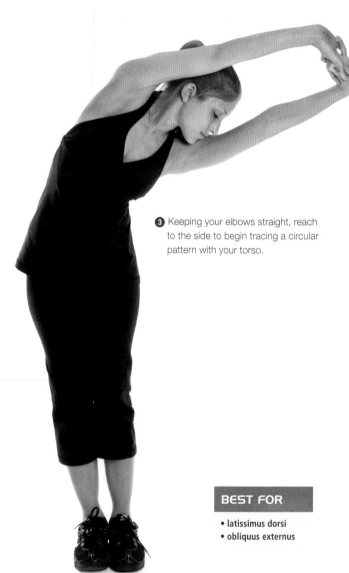

3 Keeping your elbows straight, reach to the side to begin tracing a circular pattern with your torso.

TARGETS
- Back
- Obliques

LEVEL
- Beginner

BENEFITS
- Helps correct poor posture

NOT ADVISABLE IF YOU HAVE . . .
- Lower-back pain

BEST FOR
- latissimus dorsi
- obliquus externus

4 Lean forwards and then to the opposite side as you slowly trace a full circle.

5 Return to the starting position, and then repeat the sequence three times in each direction.

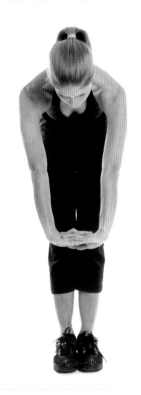

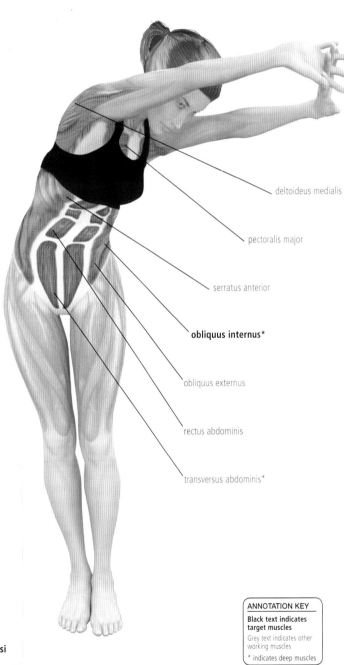

deltoideus medialis

pectoralis major

serratus anterior

obliquus internus*

obliquus externus

rectus abdominis

transversus abdominis*

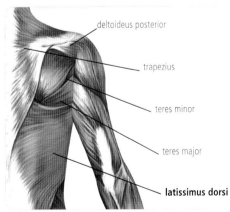

deltoideus posterior

trapezius

teres minor

teres major

latissimus dorsi

ANNOTATION KEY

Black text indicates target muscles

Grey text indicates other working muscles

* indicates deep muscles

TOE TOUCH

❶ Stand up tall, and exhale.

DO IT RIGHT
- Stack your spine one vertebra at a time.
- Connect the stretch in your back with the stretch in your hamstrings.
- Make the stretch long and smooth.

AVOID
- Tensing your neck muscles.
- Bouncing as you try to reach your hands to your toes—reach down only as far as you can comfortably extend.

TARGETS
- Spine

LEVEL
- Beginner

BENEFITS
- Stretches the spine and hamstrings
- Refines spinal stacking skills

NOT ADVISABLE IF YOU HAVE . . .
- Lower-back pain that radiates down the leg

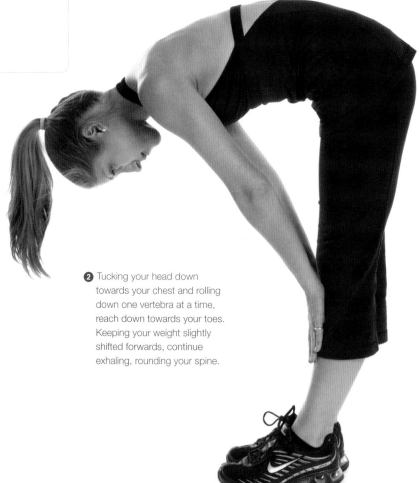

❷ Tucking your head down towards your chest and rolling down one vertebra at a time, reach down towards your toes. Keeping your weight slightly shifted forwards, continue exhaling, rounding your spine.

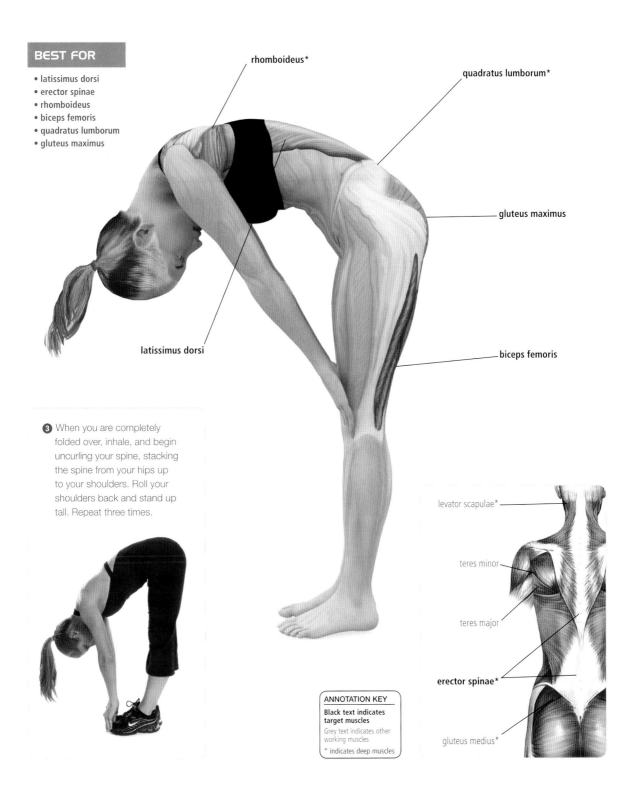

BEST FOR

- latissimus dorsi
- erector spinae
- rhomboideus
- biceps femoris
- quadratus lumborum
- gluteus maximus

rhomboideus*

quadratus lumborum*

gluteus maximus

latissimus dorsi

biceps femoris

3 When you are completely folded over, inhale, and begin uncurling your spine, stacking the spine from your hips up to your shoulders. Roll your shoulders back and stand up tall. Repeat three times.

levator scapulae*

teres minor

teres major

erector spinae*

gluteus medius*

ANNOTATION KEY

Black text indicates target muscles

Grey text indicates other working muscles

* indicates deep muscles

CAT AND DOG STRETCH

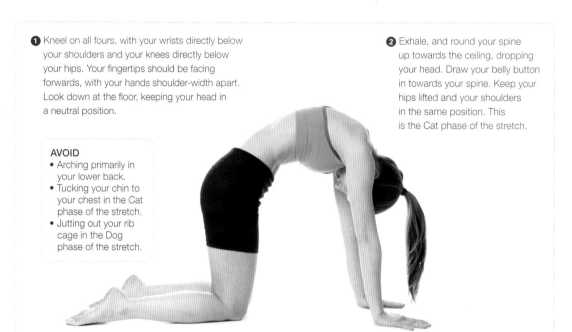

❶ Kneel on all fours, with your wrists directly below your shoulders and your knees directly below your hips. Your fingertips should be facing forwards, with your hands shoulder-width apart. Look down at the floor, keeping your head in a neutral position.

AVOID
- Arching primarily in your lower back.
- Tucking your chin to your chest in the Cat phase of the stretch.
- Jutting out your rib cage in the Dog phase of the stretch.

❷ Exhale, and round your spine up towards the ceiling, dropping your head. Draw your belly button in towards your spine. Keep your hips lifted and your shoulders in the same position. This is the Cat phase of the stretch.

TARGETS
- Lower- and middle-back extensors
- Abdominals
- Obliques

LEVEL
- Beginner

BENEFITS
- Stretches chest, shoulders, neck, spine and abdominals
- Improves range of motion

NOT ADVISABLE IF YOU HAVE . . .
- Knee injury
- Wrist pain

❸ Inhale, and uncurl your spine. Remain on your hands and knees.

❹ With your next inhalation, arch your spine, lifting your chest forwards and your tailbone towards the ceiling. Look forwards. This is the Dog phase of the stretch.

❺ Exhale, and return to a neutral position on your hands and knees.

❻ Repeat the entire sequence 10 to 20 times.

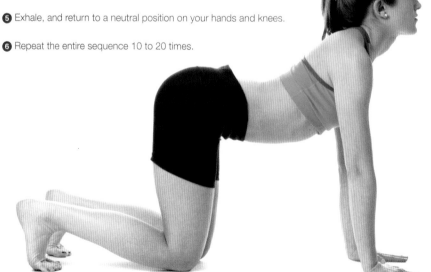

BEST FOR

• **erector spinae**

ANNOTATION KEY

Bold text indicates target muscles

Grey text indicates other working muscles

Italics indicates ligaments

* indicates deep muscles

DO IT RIGHT

• Stretch slowly and with control.
• Keep your hands and feet planted throughout the stretch.
• Lift your chin while your spine is arched.
• Start the movement of your spine in your tailbone.

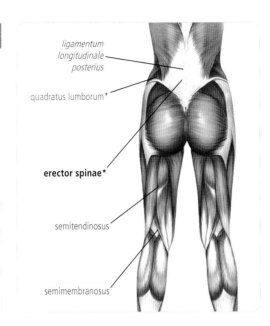

ligamentum longitudinale posterius

quadratus lumborum*

erector spinae*

semitendinosus

semimembranosus

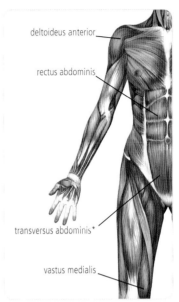

deltoideus anterior

rectus abdominis

transversus abdominis*

vastus medialis

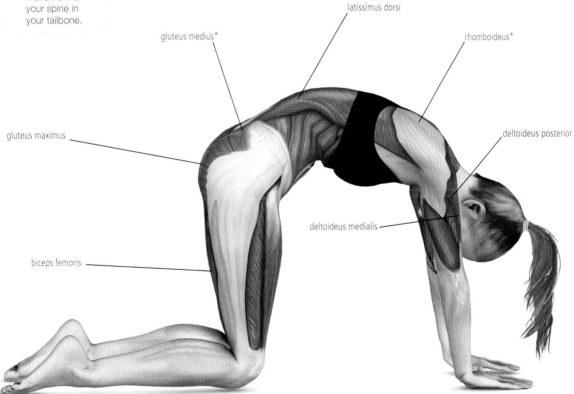

latissimus dorsi

gluteus medius*

rhomboideus*

gluteus maximus

deltoideus posterior

biceps femoris

deltoideus medialis

PIRIFORMIS STRETCH

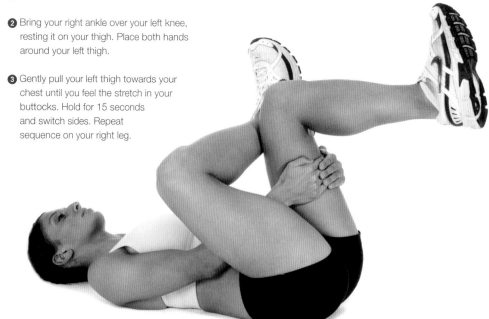

1 Lie on your back with your knees bent.

2 Bring your right ankle over your left knee, resting it on your thigh. Place both hands around your left thigh.

3 Gently pull your left thigh towards your chest until you feel the stretch in your buttocks. Hold for 15 seconds and switch sides. Repeat sequence on your right leg.

TARGETS
• Gluteal muscles

LEVEL
• Beginner

BENEFITS
• Stretches the glutes

NOT ADVISABLE IF YOU HAVE . . .
• Hip dysfunction

BEST FOR

• piriformis
• gluteus maximus
• gluteus medius
• gluteus minimus

DO IT RIGHT
• Relax your hips so that you can go deeper into the stretch.
• Perform the stretch slowly.
• Keep your head and shoulders on the floor.

AVOID
• Pulling your leg inwards too quickly.
• Twisting your lower body—instead keep your hips square.

ANNOTATION KEY

Black text indicates target muscles

Grey text indicates other working muscles

* indicates deep muscles

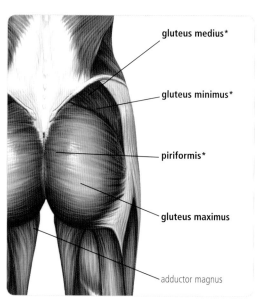

gluteus medius*

gluteus minimus*

piriformis*

gluteus maximus

adductor magnus

HIP STRETCH

BEST FOR

- adductor longus
- iliopsoas
- rhomboideus
- sternocleidomastoideus
- latissimus dorsi
- obliquus internus
- obliquus externus
- quadratus lumborum
- erector spinae
- multifidus spinae
- tractus iliotibialis
- gluteus maximus
- gluteus medius
- piriformis

1 Sit with your left leg extended straight in front of you, and bend your right knee. Cross your bent knee over the straight leg, and keep your foot flat on the floor.

2 Wrap your left arm around the bent knee so that you are able to apply pressure to your leg to rotate your torso. Place your right hand on the floor for stability.

3 Keeping your hips aligned, rotate your upper spine as you pull your chest in towards your knee.

4 Hold for 30 seconds. Slowly release, and repeat five times on each side.

DO IT RIGHT
- Keep your neck and shoulders relaxed.
- Apply even pressure to your leg with your active hand.
- Keep torso upright as you pull your knee and torso together.

AVOID
- Rounding your torso.
- Lifting the foot of your bent leg off the floor.
- Straining your neck as you rotate.

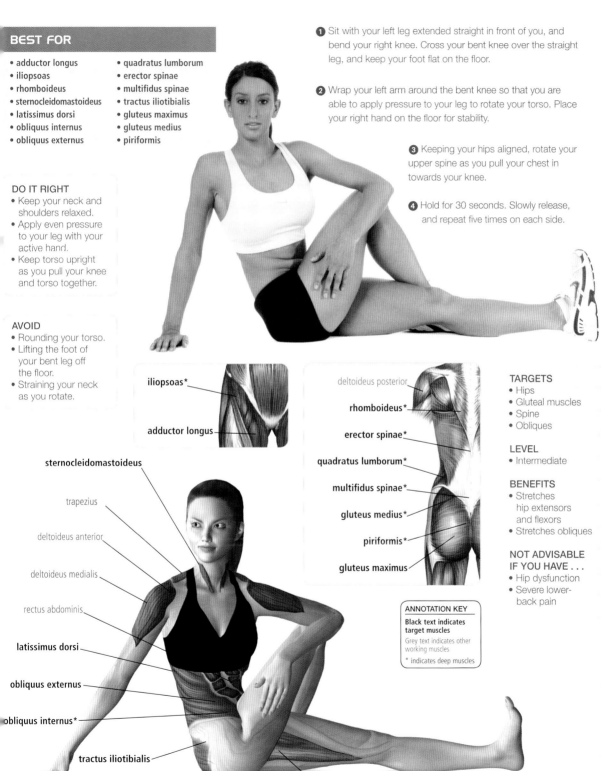

iliopsoas*
adductor longus

sternocleidomastoideus
trapezius
deltoideus anterior
deltoideus medialis
rectus abdominis
latissimus dorsi
obliquus externus
obliquus internus*
tractus iliotibialis
adductor magnus

deltoideus posterior
rhomboideus*
erector spinae*
quadratus lumborum*
multifidus spinae*
gluteus medius*
piriformis*
gluteus maximus

TARGETS
- Hips
- Gluteal muscles
- Spine
- Obliques

LEVEL
- Intermediate

BENEFITS
- Stretches hip extensors and flexors
- Stretches obliques

NOT ADVISABLE IF YOU HAVE . . .
- Hip dysfunction
- Severe lower-back pain

ANNOTATION KEY
Black text indicates target muscles
Grey text indicates other working muscles
* indicates deep muscles

HIP-TO-THIGH STRETCH

1 Kneeling on your left knee, place your right foot on the floor in front of you so that your right knee is bent less than 90 degrees.

2 Bring your torso forwards, bending your right knee so that your knee shifts towards your toes. Keeping your torso in neutral position, press your right hip forwards and downward to create a stretch over the front of your thigh. Raise your arms up towards the ceiling, keeping your shoulders relaxed.

3 Bring your arms down and move your hips backwards. Straighten your right leg, and bring your torso forwards. Place your hands on either side of your straight leg for support.

4 Hold for 10 seconds, and repeat the forwards and backwards movement five times on each leg.

DO IT RIGHT
• Keep your shoulders and neck relaxed.
• Move your entire body as one unit as you go into the stretch.

AVOID
• Extending your front knee too far over the planted foot.
• Rotating your hips.
• Shifting your back knee outwards.

TARGETS
• Hip flexors
• Hip extensors
• Hamstrings
• Quadriceps

LEVEL
• Intermediate

BENEFITS
• Stretches hips and thighs

NOT ADVISABLE IF YOU HAVE . . .
• Neck pain
• Lower-back pain

MODIFICATION
Harder: During the backwards movement, raise your back knee off the floor and straighten your back leg. Keep your hands on the floor.

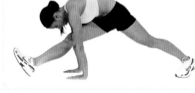

BEST FOR
• iliopsoas
• biceps femoris
• rectus femoris

obliquus externus

pectineus*

iliopsoas*

adductor longus

tensor fasciae latae

vastus intermedius*

rectus femoris

adductor magnus

vastus medialis

gracilis*

semimembranosus

biceps femoris

semitendinosus

vastus lateralis

ANNOTATION KEY
Black text indicates target muscles
Grey text indicates other working muscles
* indicates deep muscles

SPINE STRETCH

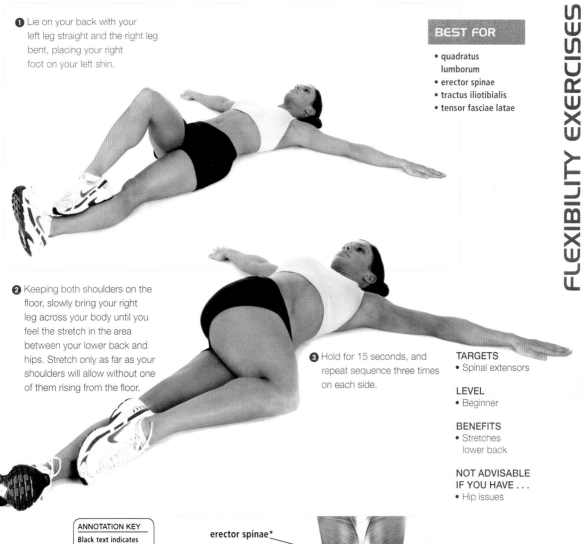

❶ Lie on your back with your left leg straight and the right leg bent, placing your right foot on your left shin.

❷ Keeping both shoulders on the floor, slowly bring your right leg across your body until you feel the stretch in the area between your lower back and hips. Stretch only as far as your shoulders will allow without one of them rising from the floor.

❸ Hold for 15 seconds, and repeat sequence three times on each side.

BEST FOR

- quadratus lumborum
- erector spinae
- tractus iliotibialis
- tensor fasciae latae

TARGETS
- Spinal extensors

LEVEL
- Beginner

BENEFITS
- Stretches lower back

NOT ADVISABLE IF YOU HAVE . . .
- Hip issues

ANNOTATION KEY

Black text indicates target muscles

Grey text indicates other working muscles

* indicates deep muscles

AVOID
- Allowing your shoulders to lift off the floor.

DO IT RIGHT
- Keep your lower back relaxed.

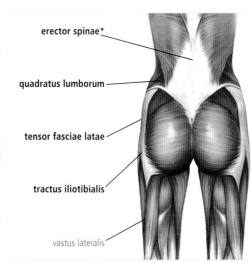

erector spinae*

quadratus lumborum

tensor fasciae latae

tractus iliotibialis

vastus lateralis

SWISS BALL HIP CROSSOVER

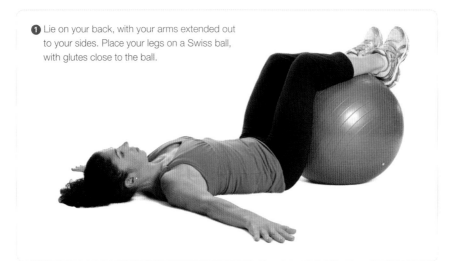

1 Lie on your back, with your arms extended out to your sides. Place your legs on a Swiss ball, with glutes close to the ball.

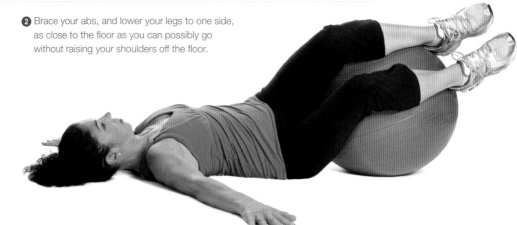

2 Brace your abs, and lower your legs to one side, as close to the floor as you can possibly go without raising your shoulders off the floor.

TARGETS
• Lower back
• Obliques

LEVEL
• Intermediate

BENEFITS
• Helps to strengthen and tone abs
• Improves core stabilisation

NOT ADVISABLE IF YOU HAVE . . .
• Lower-back issues

AVOID
• Swinging your legs too quickly; instead, try to keep the movement smooth and controlled.

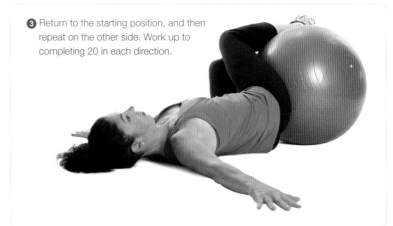

3 Return to the starting position, and then repeat on the other side. Work up to completing 20 in each direction.

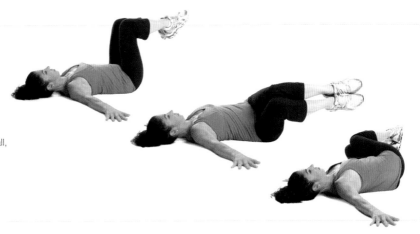

MODIFICATION

Easier: Begin with your legs lifted and bent at a 90-degree angle. Try to keep your upper body as stable as possible as you perform the crossover without the ball, alternating sides.

BEST FOR

- erector spinae
- obliquus externus

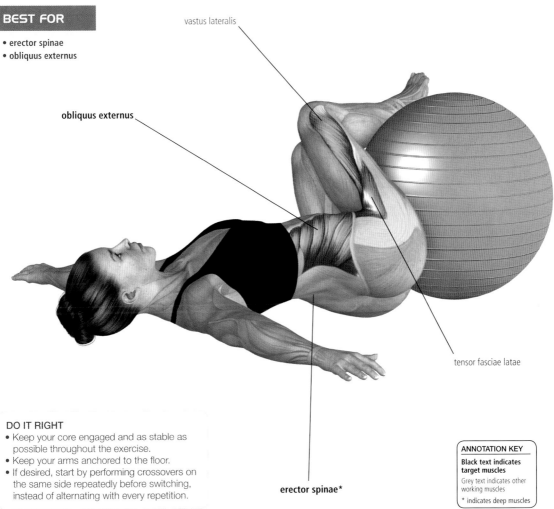

vastus lateralis

obliquus externus

tensor fasciae latae

erector spinae*

DO IT RIGHT

- Keep your core engaged and as stable as possible throughout the exercise.
- Keep your arms anchored to the floor.
- If desired, start by performing crossovers on the same side repeatedly before switching, instead of alternating with every repetition.

ANNOTATION KEY

Black text indicates target muscles

Grey text indicates other working muscles

* indicates deep muscles

KNEE-TO-CHEST HUG

❶ Lie supine on a mat with your legs together and arms outstretched.

❷ Bend your right knee, and bring your foot to your body's midline while clasping your hands together to hold your knee. Hold the stretch for 15 seconds.

TARGETS
• Lower back
• Hips

LEVEL
• Beginner

BENEFITS
• Stretches lower back, hip extensors and hip rotators

NOT ADVISABLE IF YOU HAVE . . .
• Advanced degenerative joint disease

❸ Return to the starting position.

❹ Again, clasping your hands together to hold your knee, bend your right knee, but this time rotate the right leg to the left, bringing the side of your leg against your chest.

❺ Hold the stretch for 15 seconds, and then return to the starting position. Repeat the entire sequence with the left leg bent.

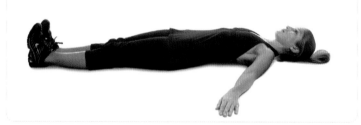

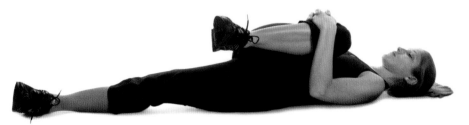

MODIFICATION

Similar level of difficulty: Follow step 1, and then draw both legs to your chest.

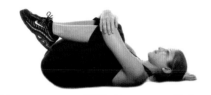

BEST FOR

- erector spinae
- latissimus dorsi
- gluteus maximus
- gluteus minimus
- piriformis
- gemellus superior
- gemellus inferior
- obturator externus
- obturator internus
- quadratus femoris

AVOID

- Lifting your buttocks off the floor.

DO IT RIGHT

- Keep your spine in neutral position.

ANNOTATION KEY

Black text indicates target muscles

Grey text indicates other working muscles

* indicates deep muscles

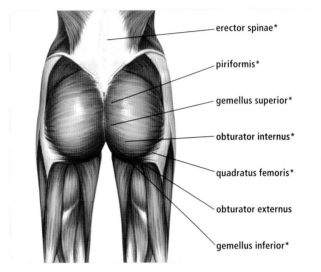

erector spinae*

piriformis*

gemellus superior*

obturator internus*

quadratus femoris*

obturator externus

gemellus inferior*

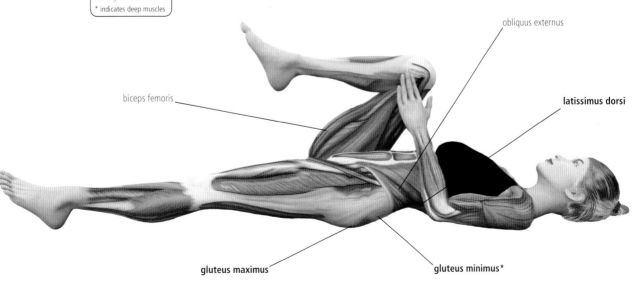

obliquus externus

biceps femoris

latissimus dorsi

gluteus maximus

gluteus minimus*

ILIOTIBIAL BAND STRETCH

① Standing, cross your left leg in front of your right.

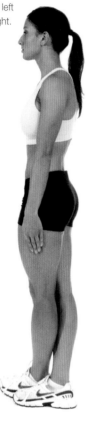

BEST FOR

- tractus iliotibialis
- biceps femoris
- gluteus maximus
- vastus lateralis

TARGETS
- Iliotibial band
- Hamstrings

LEVEL
- Beginner

BENEFITS
- Helps to stabilise knee joints
- Helps to keep hips flexible
- Stretches back, hamstrings and calves

NOT ADVISABLE IF YOU HAVE . . .
- Neck issues
- Lower-back pain

② Bend forwards from the hips while keeping both legs straight, and reach your hands towards the floor.

③ Hold for 15 seconds. Repeat the sequence three times on each leg.

AVOID
- Raising your back heel off the floor.
- Arching or rounding your back.

DO IT RIGHT
- Keep both feet flat on the floor.
- Stretch with good alignment so that your back leg and your spine form a straight line.

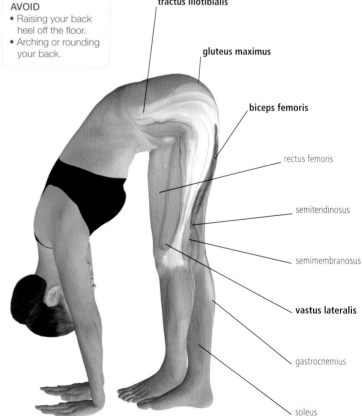

tractus iliotibialis

gluteus maximus

biceps femoris

rectus femoris

semitendinosus

semimembranosus

vastus lateralis

gastrocnemius

soleus

ANNOTATION KEY
Black text indicates target muscles
Grey text indicates other working muscles

QUADRICEPS STRETCH

BEST FOR

- rectus femoris
- vastus lateralis
- vastus medialis
- vastus intermedius

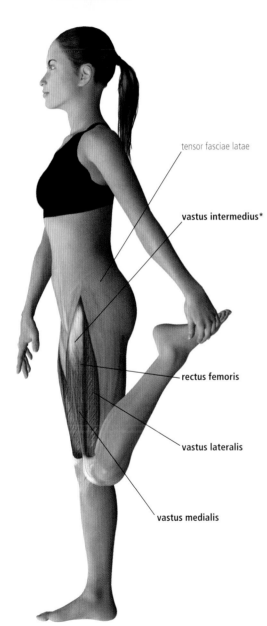

- tensor fasciae latae
- **vastus intermedius***
- **rectus femoris**
- **vastus lateralis**
- **vastus medialis**

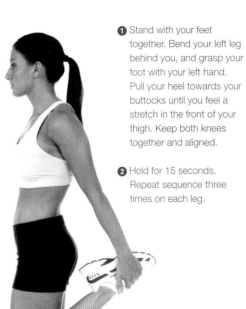

1 Stand with your feet together. Bend your left leg behind you, and grasp your foot with your left hand. Pull your heel towards your buttocks until you feel a stretch in the front of your thigh. Keep both knees together and aligned.

2 Hold for 15 seconds. Repeat sequence three times on each leg.

TARGETS
- Quadriceps

LEVEL
- Beginner

BENEFITS
- Helps to keep thigh muscles flexible

NOT ADVISABLE IF YOU HAVE . . .
- Knee issues

DO IT RIGHT
- Both knees to remain pressed together.

AVOID
- Leaning forwards with your chest.

ANNOTATION KEY
Black text indicates target muscles
Grey text indicates other working muscles

STANDING HAMSTRINGS STRETCH

1 Stand with one leg bent and the other extended in front of you with the heel on the floor.

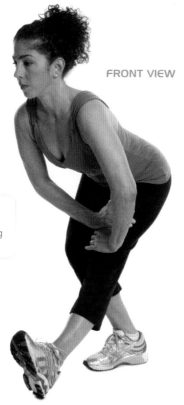

FRONT VIEW

BEST FOR
- biceps femoris
- semitendinosus
- semimembranosus

BACK VIEW

DO IT RIGHT
- Keep your front leg straight.
- Flex the foot of your front leg as you stretch.

TARGETS
- Hamstrings

LEVEL
- Beginner

BENEFITS
- Helps to keep hamstring muscles flexible

NOT ADVISABLE IF YOU HAVE . . .
- Lower-back issues
- Knee issues

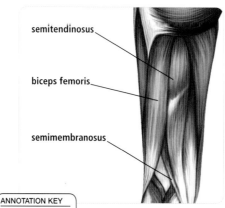

semitendinosus

biceps femoris

semimembranosus

ANNOTATION KEY
Bold text indicates target muscles
---

2 Lean over your extended leg, resting both hands above your knee. Place the majority of your body weight on your front heel while feeling the stretch in the back of your thigh. Hold for 30 seconds.

3 Switch sides and repeat. Complete three 30-second holds on each leg.

AVOID
- Allowing your back to round forwards.
- Hunching your shoulders.

STANDING CALF STRETCH

1 Stand with one foot in front of the other, with the front leg bent. With a straight back, lean over your front leg, resting both hands above the knee.

2 Place the majority of your body weight on your front heel as you feel the stretch in the calf muscle of your back leg. Hold for 30 seconds.

3 Switch sides and repeat. Complete three 30-second holds per leg.

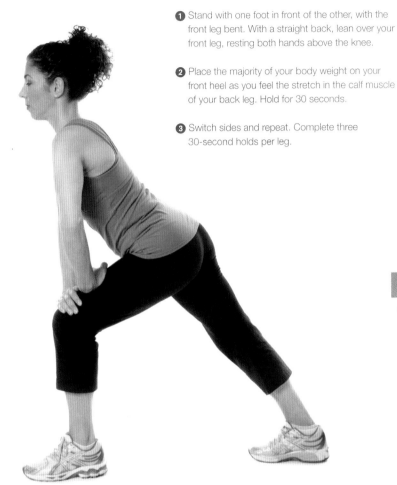

BEST FOR

• gastrocnemius

TARGETS
• Calves

LEVEL
• Intermediate

BENEFITS
• Helps to keep calf muscles flexible

AVOID IF YOU HAVE . . .
• Knee issues

DO IT RIGHT
• Keep both feet flat on the floor.
• Stretch with good alignment so that your back leg and your spine form a straight line.

AVOID
• Raising your back heel off the floor.
• Arching or rounding your back.

ANNOTATION KEY

Black text indicates target muscles
Grey text indicates other working muscles
Italics indicates tendons

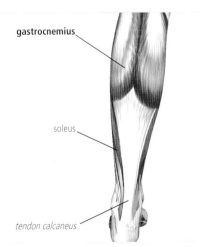

gastrocnemius

soleus

tendon calcaneus

CHILD'S POSE

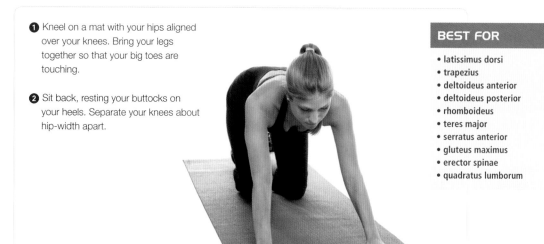

❶ Kneel on a mat with your hips aligned over your knees. Bring your legs together so that your big toes are touching.

❷ Sit back, resting your buttocks on your heels. Separate your knees about hip-width apart.

BEST FOR

- latissimus dorsi
- trapezius
- deltoideus anterior
- deltoideus posterior
- rhomboideus
- teres major
- serratus anterior
- gluteus maximus
- erector spinae
- quadratus lumborum

DO IT RIGHT
- Round your back to create a dome shape.

TARGETS
- Lower back

LEVEL
- Beginner

BENEFITS
- Stretches and relaxes the back

NOT ADVISABLE IF YOU HAVE . . .
- Knee injury

❸ Lower your chest onto your thighs as you extend your hands in front of your head, elongating your neck and spine as you stretch your tailbone towards the mat.

❹ Place your forehead on the mat, and hold this position for 30 seconds to 3 minutes.

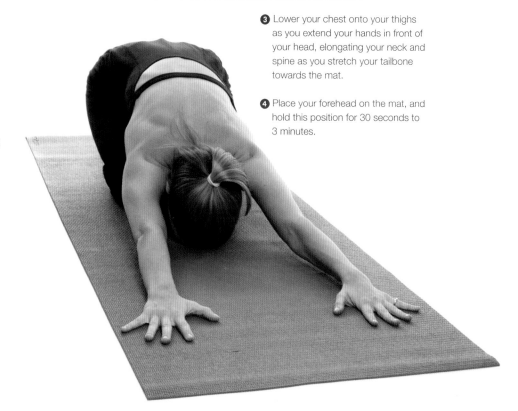

AVOID
- Rushing through the exercise. It can take a few minutes to allow your body to deepen into the full stretch.
- Compressing the back of your neck.

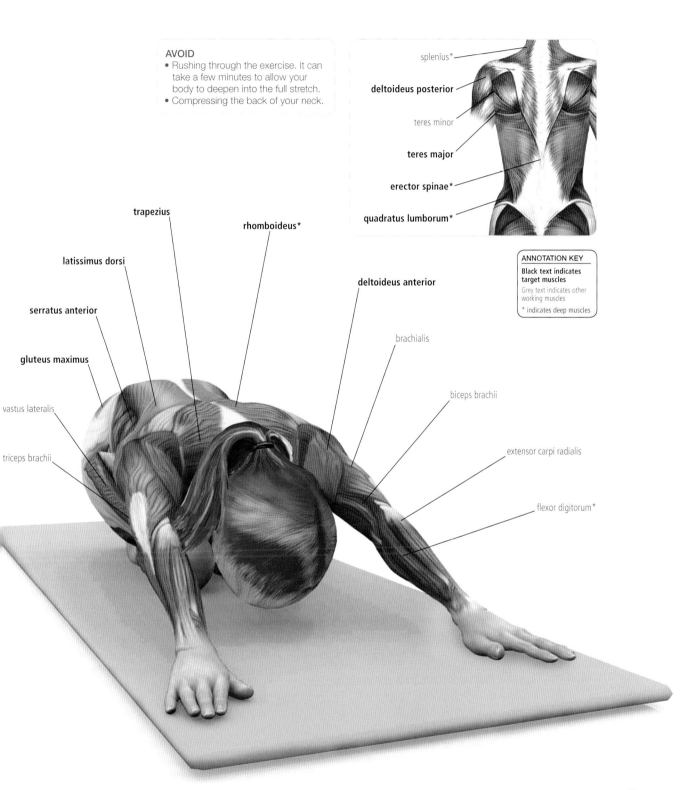

splenius*

deltoideus posterior

teres minor

teres major

erector spinae*

quadratus lumborum*

ANNOTATION KEY
Black text indicates target muscles
Grey text indicates other working muscles
* indicates deep muscles

trapezius

rhomboideus*

latissimus dorsi

deltoideus anterior

serratus anterior

brachialis

gluteus maximus

biceps brachii

vastus lateralis

extensor carpi radialis

triceps brachii

flexor digitorum*

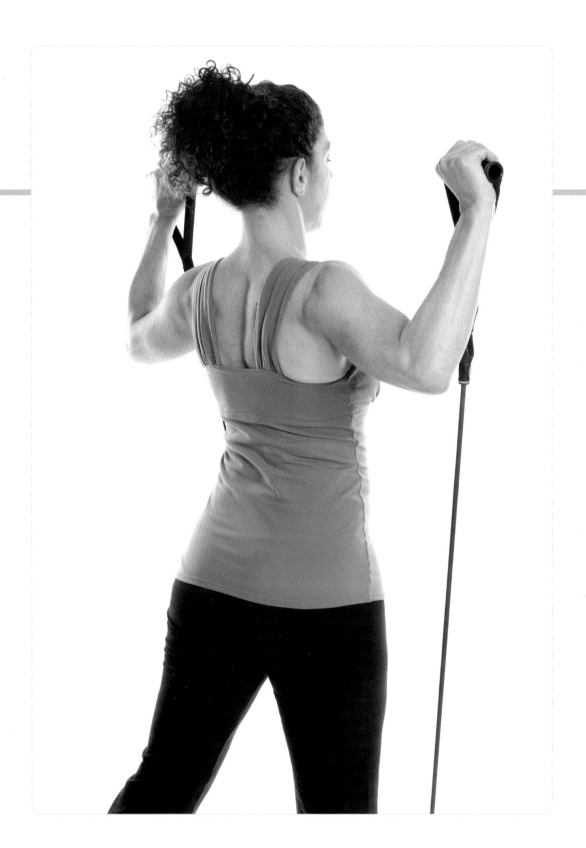

UPPER-BODY EXERCISES

We'd all like great-looking arms. Toned arms make you look younger and stronger, and allow you to move freely without worrying about any embarrassing jiggling. For sleek, shapely arms that you'll want to show off in tank tops and strapless dresses, focus on exercises that work your deltoids, biceps and triceps. Also included in this section are exercises that target other upper-body muscles, especially the upper back and chest. Upper-back exercises define and enhance the shape of your neck and shoulders, and reduce any unsightly back fat—those bulges above and below your bra strap. Exercises that tone the chest muscles (the major and minor pectorals) have another major perk: they work as natural breast lifts, giving you a more youthful, fitter silhouette.

CHAIR DIP

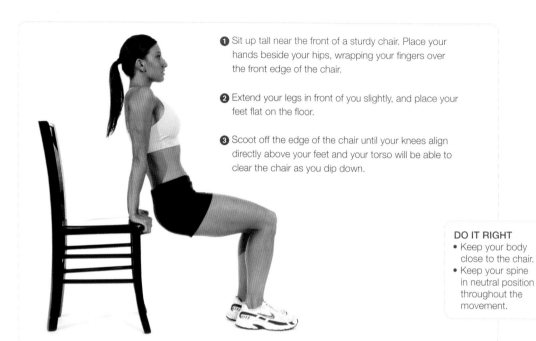

❶ Sit up tall near the front of a sturdy chair. Place your hands beside your hips, wrapping your fingers over the front edge of the chair.

❷ Extend your legs in front of you slightly, and place your feet flat on the floor.

❸ Scoot off the edge of the chair until your knees align directly above your feet and your torso will be able to clear the chair as you dip down.

DO IT RIGHT
• Keep your body close to the chair.
• Keep your spine in neutral position throughout the movement.

TARGETS
• Triceps
• Shoulder and core stabilisers

LEVEL
• Intermediate

BENEFITS
• Strengthens the shoulder girdle
• Trains the torso to remain stable while the legs and arms are in motion

NOT ADVISABLE IF YOU HAVE . . .
• Shoulder pain
• Wrist pain

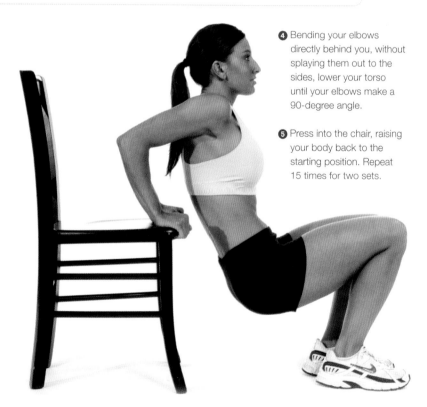

❹ Bending your elbows directly behind you, without splaying them out to the sides, lower your torso until your elbows make a 90-degree angle.

❺ Press into the chair, raising your body back to the starting position. Repeat 15 times for two sets.

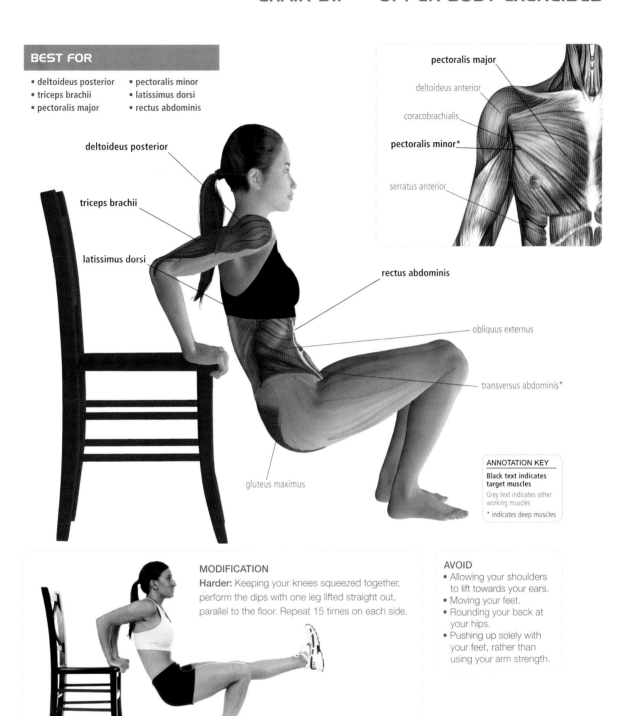

BEST FOR

- deltoideus posterior
- triceps brachii
- pectoralis major
- pectoralis minor
- latissimus dorsi
- rectus abdominis

deltoideus posterior

triceps brachii

latissimus dorsi

gluteus maximus

pectoralis major

deltoideus anterior

coracobrachialis

pectoralis minor*

serratus anterior

rectus abdominis

obliquus externus

transversus abdominis*

ANNOTATION KEY

Black text indicates target muscles

Grey text indicates other working muscles

* indicates deep muscles

MODIFICATION

Harder: Keeping your knees squeezed together, perform the dips with one leg lifted straight out, parallel to the floor. Repeat 15 times on each side.

AVOID

- Allowing your shoulders to lift towards your ears.
- Moving your feet.
- Rounding your back at your hips.
- Pushing up solely with your feet, rather than using your arm strength.

45

CHAIR CRUNCH

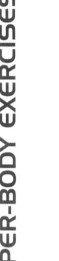

❶ Sit up tall on a chair with your hands grasping the sides of the seat and your arms straight.

❷ Step forwards so that your knees are bent but your buttocks are lifted off the chair. Your hips and knees should be bent to form 90-degree angles.

DO IT RIGHT
• Keep your spine in neutral position as you progress through the motion.
• Align your knees over your ankles.
• Keep your body close to the chair.

AVOID
• Allowing your shoulders to lift towards your ears.

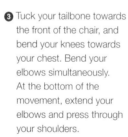

TARGETS
• Shoulders
• Upper arms
• Abdominals

LEVEL
• Advanced

BENEFITS
• Strengthens upper body
• Improves shoulder stability

NOT ADVISABLE IF YOU HAVE . . .
• Shoulder pain
• Neck pain

❸ Tuck your tailbone towards the front of the chair, and bend your knees towards your chest. Bend your elbows simultaneously. At the bottom of the movement, extend your elbows and press through your shoulders.

❹ Keeping your head in neutral position, press into the chair and lower your legs to return to the starting position. Repeat 15 times for two sets.

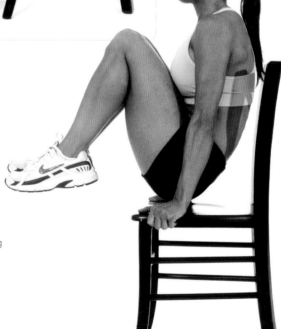

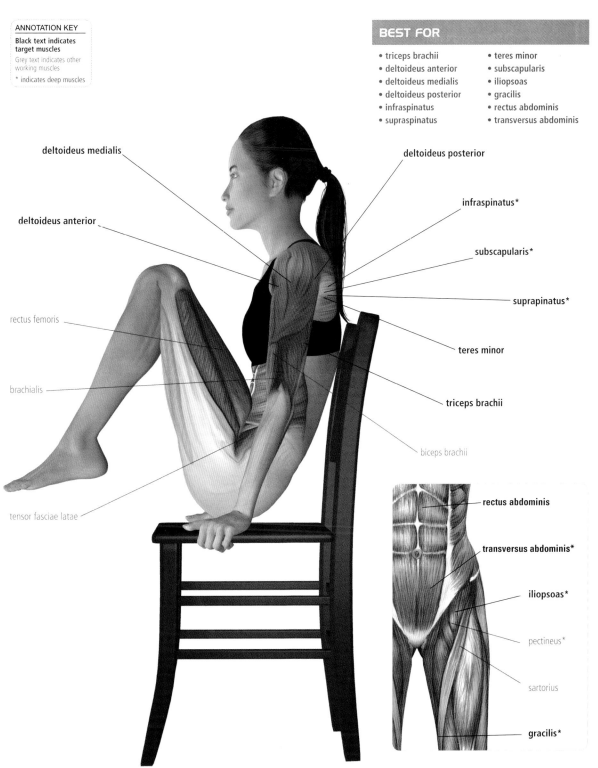

ANNOTATION KEY

Black text indicates target muscles

Grey text indicates other working muscles

* indicates deep muscles

BEST FOR

- triceps brachii
- deltoideus anterior
- deltoideus medialis
- deltoideus posterior
- infraspinatus
- supraspinatus
- teres minor
- subscapularis
- iliopsoas
- gracilis
- rectus abdominis
- transversus abdominis

deltoideus medialis

deltoideus anterior

rectus femoris

brachialis

tensor fasciae latae

deltoideus posterior

infraspinatus*

subscapularis*

suprapinatus*

teres minor

triceps brachii

biceps brachii

rectus abdominis

transversus abdominis*

iliopsoas*

pectineus*

sartorius

gracilis*

OVERHEAD PRESS

1 Stand upright with one leg extended about a foot behind you, heel off the ground. Position a resistance band beneath the foot of your front leg. Hold the handles in both hands, with arms bent, so that the resistance band is taut.

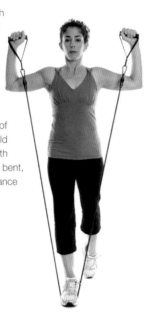

2 Straighten both arms so that they are extended to full lockout above your head a few inches in front of your shoulders.

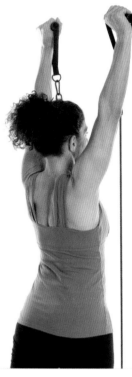

TARGETS
• Shoulders
• Triceps

LEVEL
• Beginner

BENEFITS
• Strengthens and tones shoulders and upper arms

NOT ADVISABLE IF YOU HAVE . . .
• Shoulder issues

3 Lower your arms to starting position and then repeat. Perform three sets of 15.

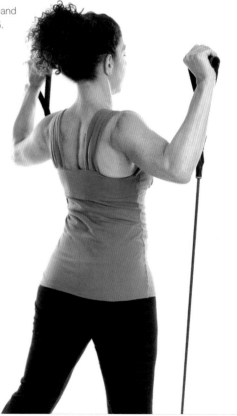

DO IT RIGHT
• Keep the rest of your body stable as you extend your arms.
• Gaze forwards throughout the exercise.
• Keep your abs engaged and pulled in.
• Extend both arms at the same time.

AVOID
• Twisting your torso.

BEST FOR
• deltoideus anterior
• triceps brachii

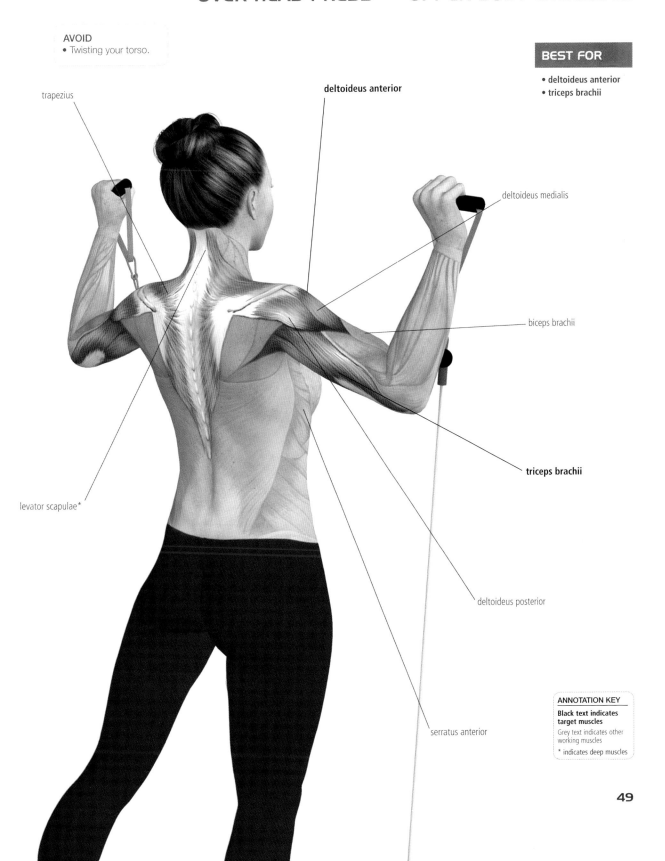

trapezius

deltoideus anterior

deltoideus medialis

biceps brachii

triceps brachii

levator scapulae*

deltoideus posterior

serratus anterior

ANNOTATION KEY

**Black text indicates
target muscles**

Grey text indicates other
working muscles

* indicates deep muscles

49

ALTERNATING CHEST PRESS

1 Run a resistance band around a sturdy, stable object, such as a pole or column. Stand facing away from the object, holding both ends of the resistance band in front of your chest.

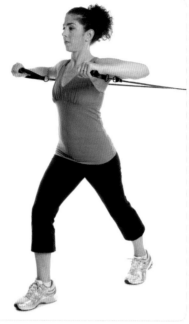

AVOID
• Twisting your torso.
• Hunching your shoulders.

2 Extend one arm straight in front of you to full lockout position, keeping the other arm steady.

3 With control, bring the arm back to starting position. Repeat with the other arm, completing three sets of 15 repetitions per arm.

TARGETS
• Chest
• Core
• Shoulders
• Triceps

LEVEL
• Beginner

BENEFITS
• Strengthens and tones pectorals
• Stabilises core

NOT ADVISABLE IF YOU HAVE . . .
• Shoulder issues

DO IT RIGHT
• Keep one arm motionless as you extend the other to lockout.
• Maintain a stable torso.
• Keep your feet in place as you extend your arm.
• Engage your abs throughout the exercise.
• Keep your arms level with your shoulders.

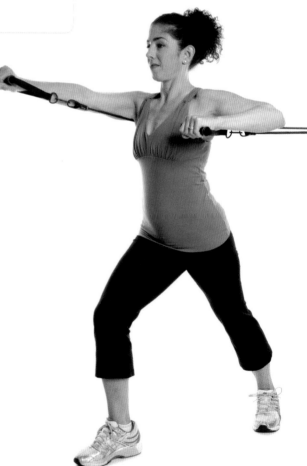

BEST FOR

• pectoralis major

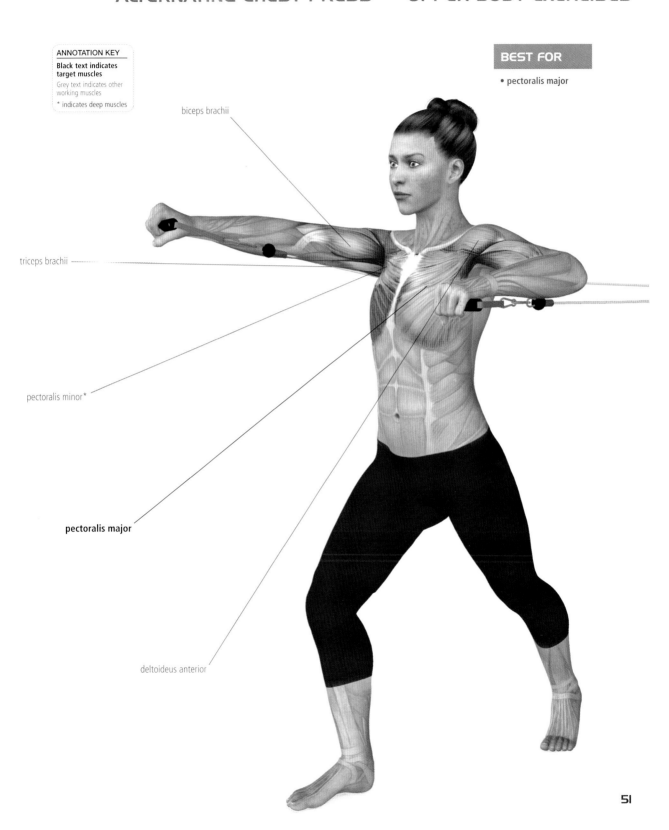

biceps brachii

triceps brachii

pectoralis minor*

pectoralis major

deltoideus anterior

STANDING FLY

① Run a resistance band around a sturdy, stable object such as a pole or column. Stand upright, with your feet planted shoulder-width apart and your knees soft. Grasp both of the handles of your resistance band, and extend your arms in front of you to almost shoulder height, holding the band taut.

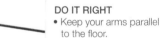

BEST FOR

• pectoralis major

TARGETS
• Back
• Chest
• Upper back

LEVEL
• Beginner

BENEFITS
• Strengthens and tones shoulders and upper back

NOT ADVISABLE IF YOU HAVE . . .
• Lower-back issues
• Shoulder pain

② Slowly and with control, bring both arms out to the sides.

③ Return to starting position and repeat. Complete three sets of 15 repetitions.

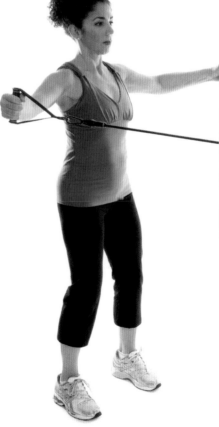

DO IT RIGHT
• Keep your arms parallel to the floor.
• Keep your back flat and your torso stable.
• Engage your abs and glutes throughout the exercise.
• Move both arms at the same time.

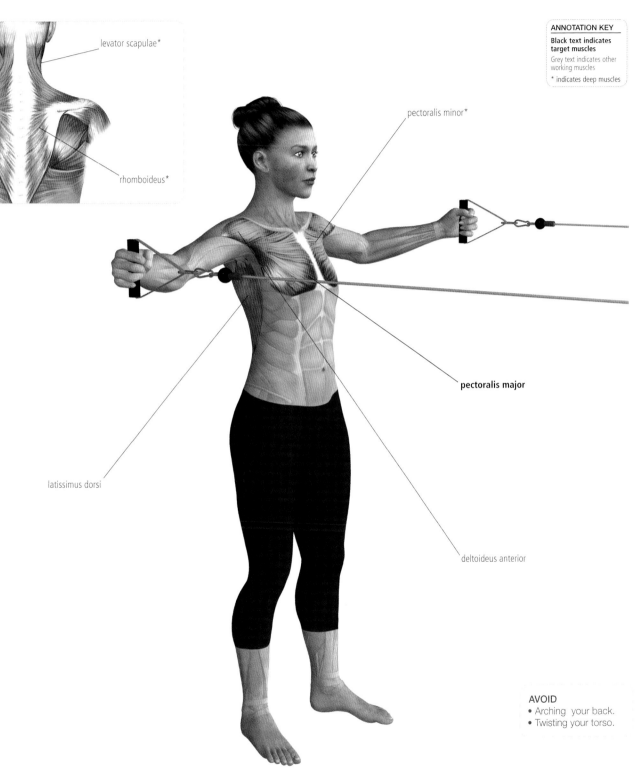

levator scapulae*

rhomboideus*

pectoralis minor*

pectoralis major

latissimus dorsi

deltoideus anterior

AVOID
• Arching your back.
• Twisting your torso.

UPWARDS PLANK

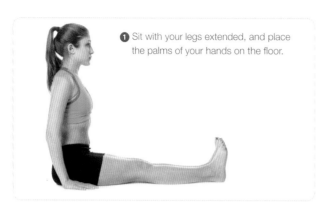

1 Sit with your legs extended, and place the palms of your hands on the floor.

DO IT RIGHT
- Use your hamstrings and shoulders to open your hips and chest, rather than overextend your back. If your hamstrings are too weak, keep your legs bent while holding the lift in your hips.
- Breathe steadily, using the breath to deepen the extension in your upper back.

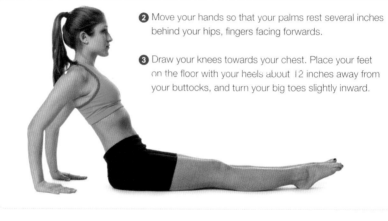

2 Move your hands so that your palms rest several inches behind your hips, fingers facing forwards.

3 Draw your knees towards your chest. Place your feet on the floor with your heels about 12 inches away from your buttocks, and turn your big toes slightly inward.

TARGETS
- Upper back
- Upper arms
- Shoulders
- Chest
- Hamstrings

LEVEL
- Intermediate

BENEFITS
- Strengthens the shoulders, spine, arms and hamstrings
- Stretches the hips and chest

NOT ADVISABLE IF YOU HAVE . . .
- Neck injury
- Wrist injury

4 Exhale, pressing down with your hands and feet and lifting your hips until your back and thighs are parallel to the floor. Your shoulders should be directly above your wrists.

5 Without lowering your hips, straighten your legs one at a time.

6 Lifting your chest and bringing your shoulder blades together, push your hips higher, creating a slight arch in your back.

7 Gently elongate your neck, and let it drop back.

8 Hold for 30 seconds, and return to a seated position.

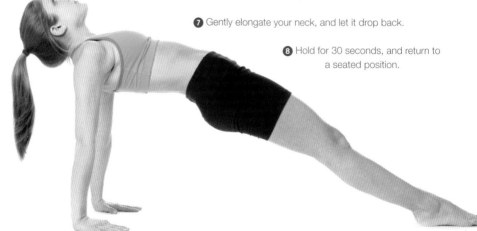

BEST FOR

- deltoideus medialis
- deltoideus anterior
- deltoideus posterior
- triceps brachii
- teres major
- teres minor
- erector spinae
- gluteus maximus
- gluteus medius
- adductor magnus
- biceps femoris
- pectoralis major

AVOID

- Squeezing your glutes to create the lift.
- Using your glutes to maintain the position.
- Allowing your hips to sag.

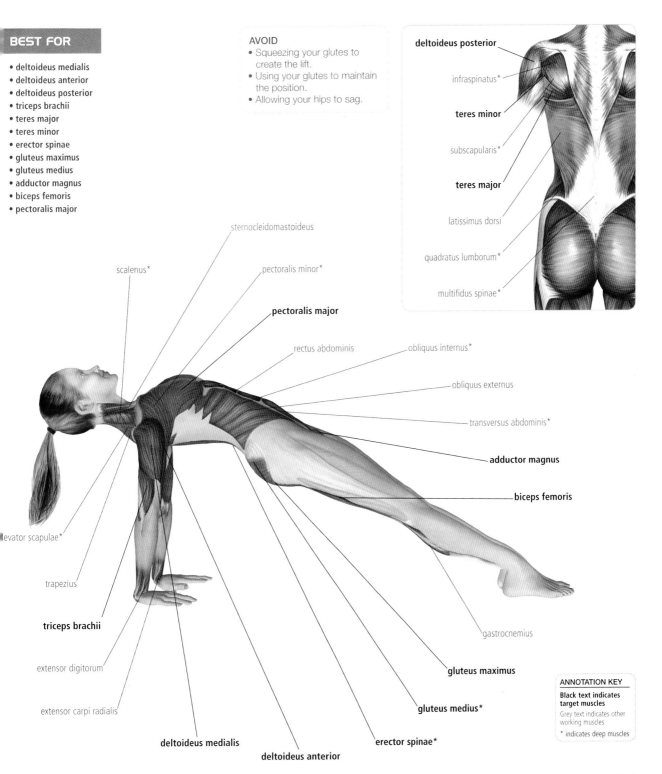

deltoideus posterior

infraspinatus*

teres minor

subscapularis*

teres major

latissimus dorsi

quadratus lumborum*

multifidus spinae*

sternocleidomastoideus

scalenus*

pectoralis minor*

pectoralis major

rectus abdominis

obliquus internus*

obliquus externus

transversus abdominis*

adductor magnus

biceps femoris

levator scapulae*

trapezius

triceps brachii

extensor digitorum

extensor carpi radialis

deltoideus medialis

deltoideus anterior

erector spinae*

gluteus medius*

gluteus maximus

gastrocnemius

ANNOTATION KEY

Black text indicates target muscles

Grey text indicates other working muscles

* indicates deep muscles

55

SWISS BALL PULLOVER

1 Lie face-up on a Swiss ball, with your upper back, neck, and head supported. Your body should be extended with your torso long, knees bent at a right angle and feet planted on the floor a little wider than shoulder-distance apart. Grasp a hand weight or dumbbell in each hand, and extend your arms behind you, level with your shoulders so that your body from knees to fingertips forms a straight line.

AVOID
- Locking your arms when they are extended behind your head.
- Arching your back.
- Rushing through the exercise.

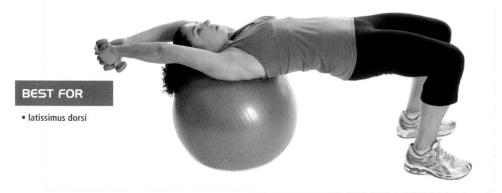

BEST FOR
- latissimus dorsi

TARGETS
- Upper back
- Core

LEVEL
- Intermediate

BENEFITS
- Strengthens upper back
- Stabilises core

NOT ADVISABLE IF YOU HAVE . . .
- Shoulder issues

2 Keeping the rest of your body stable and your arms as straight as possible, raise your arms upwards so that they are perpendicular to your body.

3 Return your arms to starting position. Repeat, performing three sets of 15 repetitions.

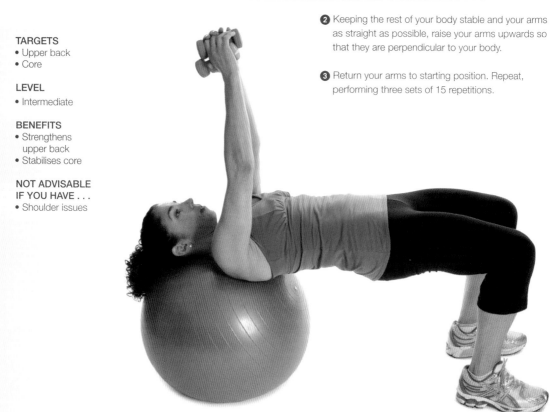

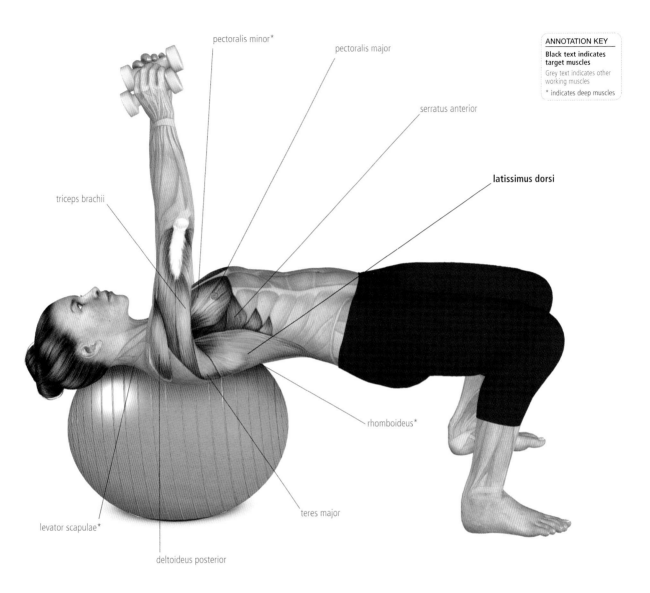

pectoralis minor*

pectoralis major

serratus anterior

latissimus dorsi

triceps brachii

ANNOTATION KEY

Black text indicates target muscles

Grey text indicates other working muscles

* indicates deep muscles

rhomboideus*

levator scapulae*

teres major

deltoideus posterior

DO IT RIGHT
- Ease into the movement.
- Keep your arms directly above your shoulders when lifting the weights overhead.
- Keep your torso stable and feet planted throughout the exercise.
- Engage your abs.
- Keep your buttocks and pelvis lifted so that your upper legs, torso and neck form a straight line.
- Move your arms smoothly and with control.

MODIFICATION
Similar level of difficulty: Instead of using hand weights, grasp a medicine ball in your hands as you perform the exercise.

SWISS BALL TRICEPS EXTENSION

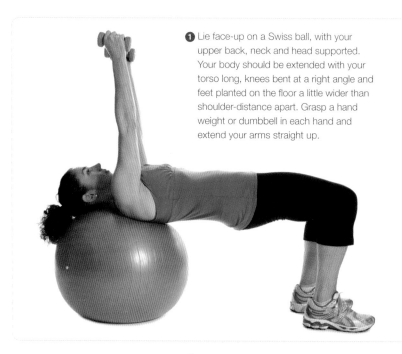

① Lie face-up on a Swiss ball, with your upper back, neck and head supported. Your body should be extended with your torso long, knees bent at a right angle and feet planted on the floor a little wider than shoulder-distance apart. Grasp a hand weight or dumbbell in each hand and extend your arms straight up.

DO IT RIGHT

- Keep your forearms stable and your elbows over your shoulders.
- Keep your torso stable and feet planted throughout the exercise.
- Engage your abs.
- Keep your glutes and pelvis lifted so that your upper legs, torso and neck form a straight line.
- Move smoothly and with control.

BEST FOR

- triceps brachii

TARGETS
- Triceps

LEVEL
- Intermediate

BENEFITS
- Strengthens and tones triceps

NOT ADVISABLE IF YOU HAVE . . .
- Elbow pain

② Bend your elbows as you lower the weights towards your head.

③ Straighten your arms upwards to starting position and then repeat. Perform three sets of 15 repetitions.

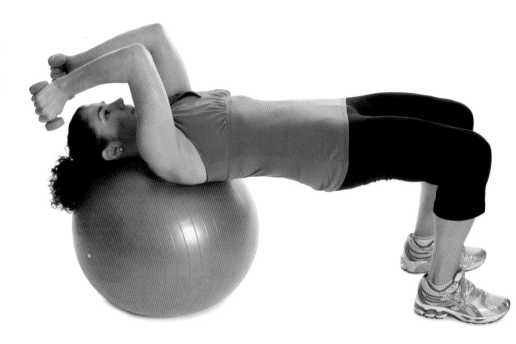

AVOID
- Arching your back.
- Flaring your elbows outward.
- Swinging your weights—especially important as the weights are close to your head.

ANNOTATION KEY

Black text indicates target muscles

Grey text indicates other working muscles

* indicates deep muscles

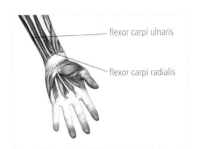

flexor carpi ulnaris

flexor carpi radialis

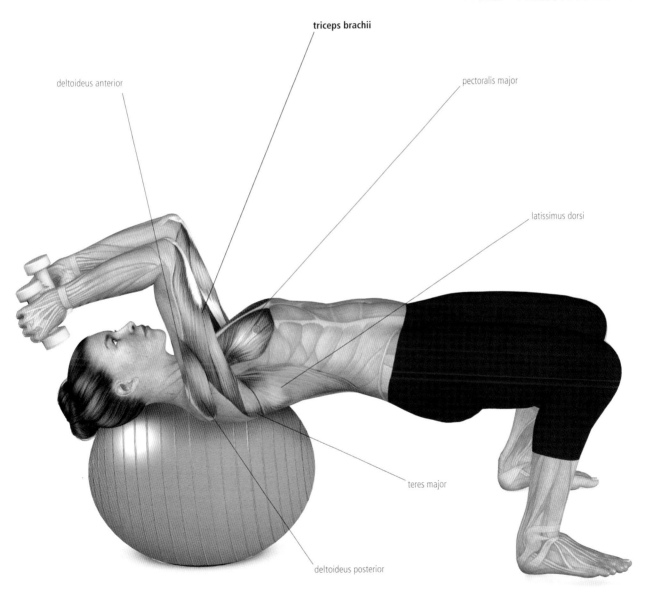

triceps brachii

deltoideus anterior

pectoralis major

latissimus dorsi

teres major

deltoideus posterior

SWISS BALL FLY

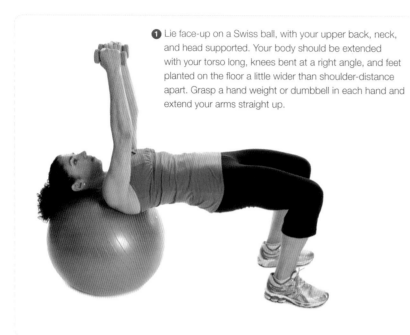

1 Lie face-up on a Swiss ball, with your upper back, neck, and head supported. Your body should be extended with your torso long, knees bent at a right angle, and feet planted on the floor a little wider than shoulder-distance apart. Grasp a hand weight or dumbbell in each hand and extend your arms straight up.

DO IT RIGHT
- When lifting the weights overhead, keep your arms directly above your shoulders.
- Keep your torso stable and feet planted throughout the exercise.
- Engage your abs.
- Keep your buttocks and pelvis lifted so that your upper legs, torso and neck form a straight line.
- Move your arms smoothly and with control.

AVOID
- Arching your back.
- Swinging your arms.

TARGETS
- Chest

LEVEL
- Beginner

BENEFITS
- Strengthens and tones pectoral muscles

NOT ADVISABLE IF YOU HAVE . . .
- Shoulder issues

2 Keeping the rest of your body stable, bring your arms to your sides.

3 Return your arms to starting position. Repeat, completing three sets of 15.

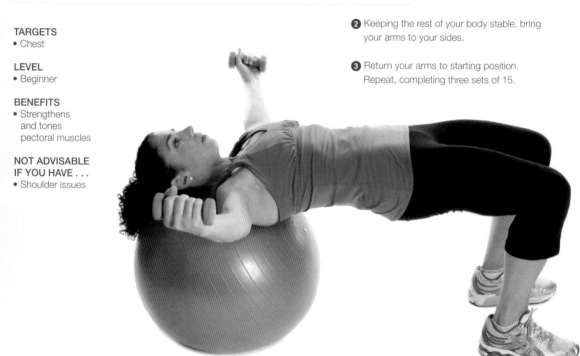

MODIFICATION

Similar level of difficulty: Instead of holding hand weights, loop a fitness band under your ball and grasp both handles. Keep your arms extended as you hold the strap taut throughout the exercise.

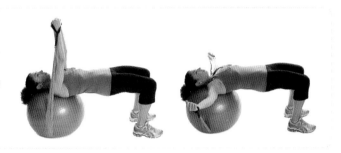

BEST FOR

• pectoralis major
• pectoralis minor

ANNOTATION KEY

Black text indicates target muscles
Grey text indicates other working muscles
* indicates deep muscles

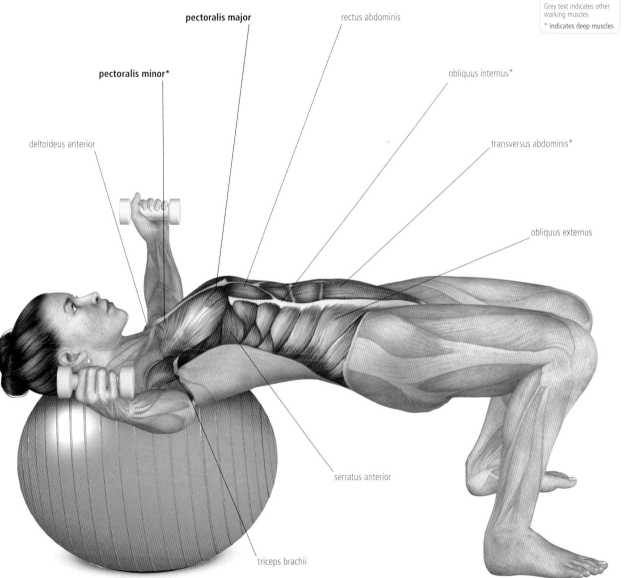

pectoralis major

rectus abdominis

pectoralis minor*

obliquus internus*

deltoideus anterior

transversus abdominis*

obliquus externus

serratus anterior

triceps brachii

61

PUSH-UP

❶ From a standing position, walk your hands out until they are directly beneath your shoulders in a high plank position.

❷ Inhale, and set your body by drawing your abdominals to your spine. Squeeze your buttocks and legs together and stretch out of your heels, bringing your body into a straight line.

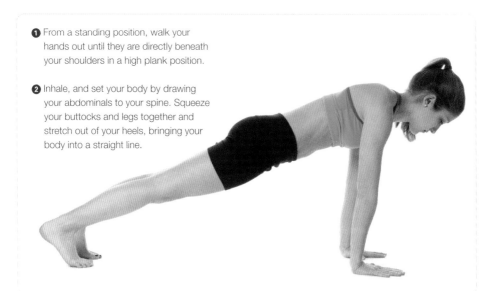

TARGETS
• Chest
• Upper arms

LEVEL
• Beginner

BENEFITS
• Strengthens the core stabilisers, shoulders, back, buttocks and pectoral muscles

NOT ADVISABLE IF YOU HAVE . . .
• Shoulder issues
• Wrist pain
• Lower-back pain

❸ Exhale and inhale as you bend your elbows and lower your body towards the floor.

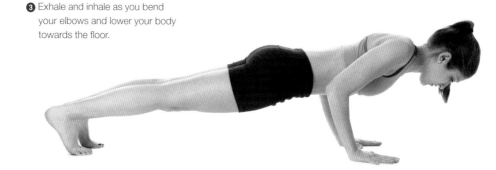

❹ Push upwards to return to plank position. Keep your elbows close to your body. Repeat eight times.

❺ Inhale as you lift your hips into the air, and walk your hands back towards your feet. Exhale slowly, rolling up one vertebra at a time into your starting position. Repeat the entire exercise three times.

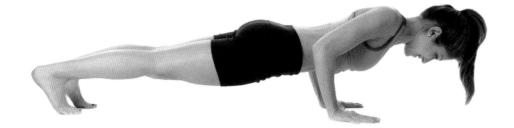

DO IT RIGHT
- Relax your neck, keeping it long as you perform the upwards movement.
- Squeeze your glutes as you scoop in your abdominals for stability.

AVOID
- Allowing your shoulders to lift towards your ears.

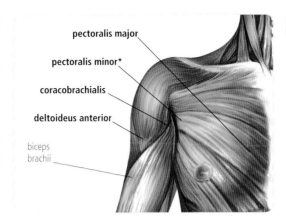

pectoralis major

pectoralis minor*

coracobrachialis

deltoideus anterior

biceps brachii

BEST FOR

- triceps brachii
- pectoralis major
- pectoralis minor
- coracobrachialis
- deltoideus anterior
- rectus abdominis
- transversus abdominis
- obliquus externus
- obliquus internus
- trapezius

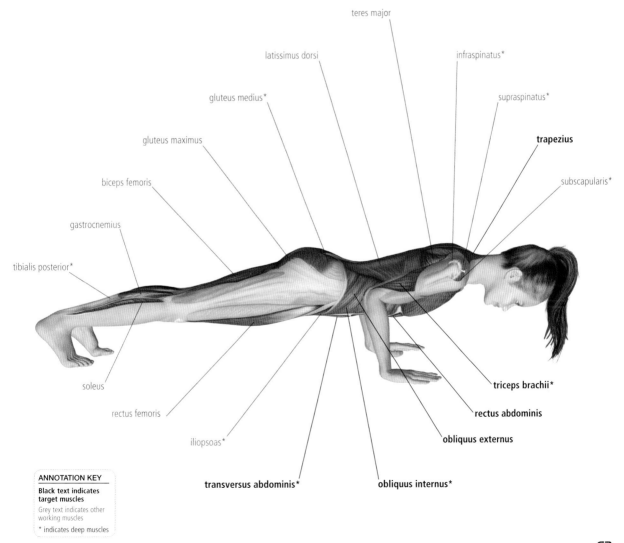

teres major

latissimus dorsi

infraspinatus*

supraspinatus*

gluteus medius*

trapezius

gluteus maximus

subscapularis*

biceps femoris

gastrocnemius

tibialis posterior*

triceps brachii*

soleus

rectus abdominis

rectus femoris

obliquus externus

iliopsoas*

transversus abdominis*

obliquus internus*

ANNOTATION KEY

Black text indicates target muscles

Grey text indicates other working muscles

* indicates deep muscles

PRONE TRUNK RAISE

❶ Lie prone on the floor. Bend your elbows, placing your hands flat on the floor on either side of your chest. Keep your elbows pulled in towards your body. Separate your legs hip-width apart, and extend through your toes. The tops of your feet should be touching the floor.

❷ Inhale, and press against the floor with your hands and the tops of your feet, lifting your torso and hips off the floor. Contract your thighs, and tuck your tailbone towards your pubis.

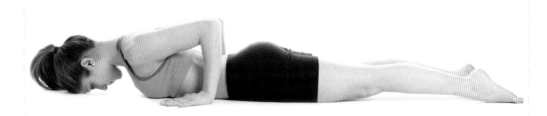

❸ Lift through the top of your chest, fully extending your arms and creating an arch in your back from your upper torso. Push your shoulders down and back, and elongate your neck as you gaze slightly upwards.

❹ Hold for 15 to 30 seconds, and exhale as you lower yourself to the floor.

TARGETS
- Upper back
- Lower back
- Upper arms
- Gluteal muscles

LEVEL
- Beginner

BENEFITS
- Strengthens spine, arms and wrists
- Stretches chest and abdominals
- Improves posture

NOT ADVISABLE IF YOU HAVE . . .
- Back injury
- Wrist injury or carpal tunnel syndrome

DO IT RIGHT
- Elongate your legs and arms to create full extension.
- Make sure that your wrists are positioned directly below your shoulders so that you don't exert too much pressure on your lower back.

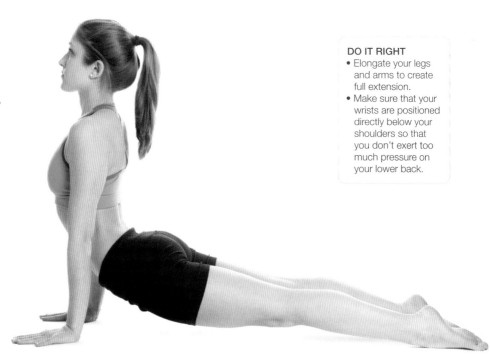

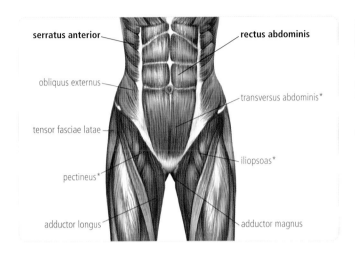

serratus anterior
rectus abdominis
obliquus externus
transversus abdominis*
tensor fasciae latae
iliopsoas*
pectineus*
adductor longus
adductor magnus

AVOID
- Lifting your shoulders up towards your ears.
- Hyperextending your elbows.
- Jutting your rib cage out of your chest.
- Dropping your thighs to the floor.

BEST FOR
- rhomboideus
- teres major
- teres minor
- trapezius
- latissimus dorsi
- erector spinae
- quadratus lumborum
- gluteus maximus
- pectoralis major
- serratus anterior
- rectus abdominis
- triceps brachii

ANNOTATION KEY

Black text indicates target muscles

Grey text indicates other working muscles

* indicates deep muscles

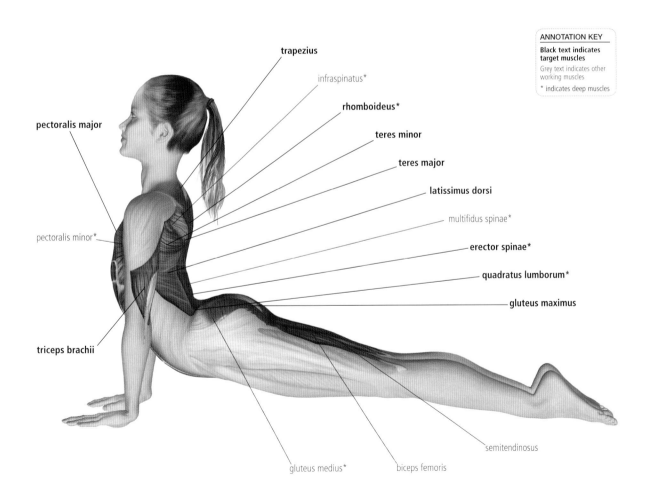

trapezius
infraspinatus*
rhomboideus*
teres minor
teres major
latissimus dorsi
multifidus spinae*
erector spinae*
quadratus lumborum*
gluteus maximus
pectoralis major
pectoralis minor*
triceps brachii
gluteus medius*
biceps femoris
semitendinosus

DUMBBELL UPRIGHT ROW

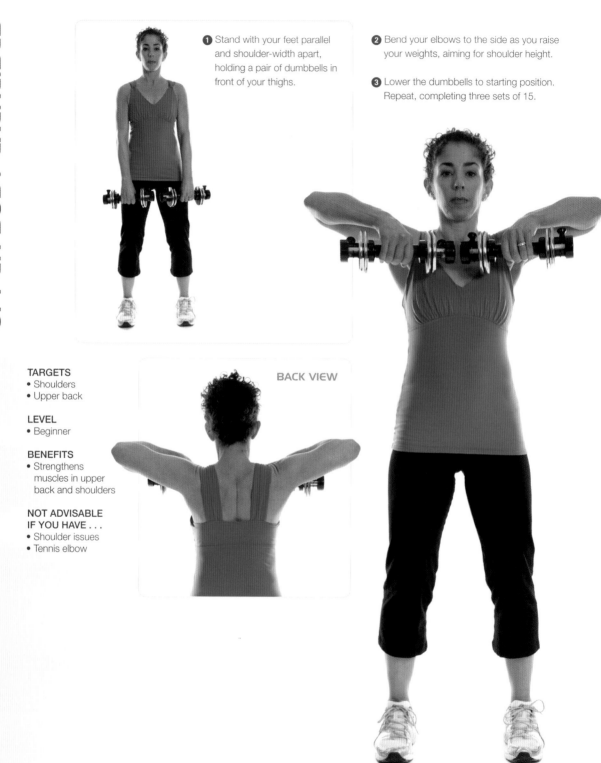

❶ Stand with your feet parallel and shoulder-width apart, holding a pair of dumbbells in front of your thighs.

❷ Bend your elbows to the side as you raise your weights, aiming for shoulder height.

❸ Lower the dumbbells to starting position. Repeat, completing three sets of 15.

BACK VIEW

TARGETS
• Shoulders
• Upper back

LEVEL
• Beginner

BENEFITS
• Strengthens muscles in upper back and shoulders

NOT ADVISABLE IF YOU HAVE . . .
• Shoulder issues
• Tennis elbow

AVOID
- Swinging your weights; instead, move slowly and with control.
- Arching your back or slumping forwards.

DO IT RIGHT
- Keep your torso stable, your back straight, and your abs engaged.
- Lead with your elbows.

ANNOTATION KEY

Black text indicates target muscles

Grey text indicates other working muscles

* indicates deep muscles

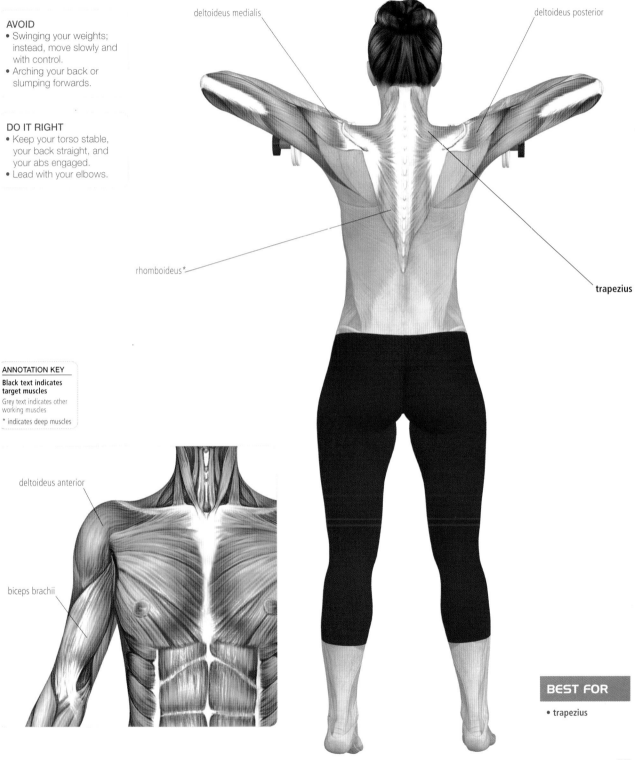

deltoideus medialis

deltoideus posterior

rhomboideus*

trapezius

deltoideus anterior

biceps brachii

BEST FOR
- trapezius

ALTERNATING DUMBBELL CURL

1 Stand upright, with your feet planted about shoulder-width apart and your knees very slightly bent. Hold a hand weight or dumbbell in each hand, with your arms down along your sides, palms facing forwards.

2 In a smooth, controlled movement, bend one arm as you raise the weight towards your shoulder.

3 As you begin to lower your arm, begin to raise the other one, and repeat on the other side. Continue to alternate, completing three sets of 15 per arm.

TARGETS
• Biceps

LEVEL
• Beginner

BENEFITS
• Strengthens and tones upper arms

NOT ADVISABLE IF YOU HAVE . . .
• Lower-back issues

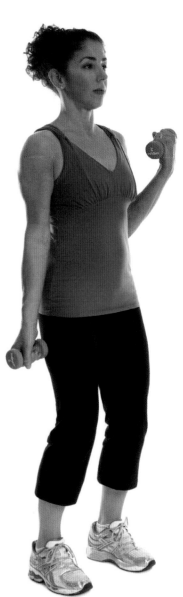

DO IT RIGHT
• Keep your knees soft throughout the exercise.
• Gaze forwards.
• Keep one arm still while the other is moving.
• Keep your torso still.

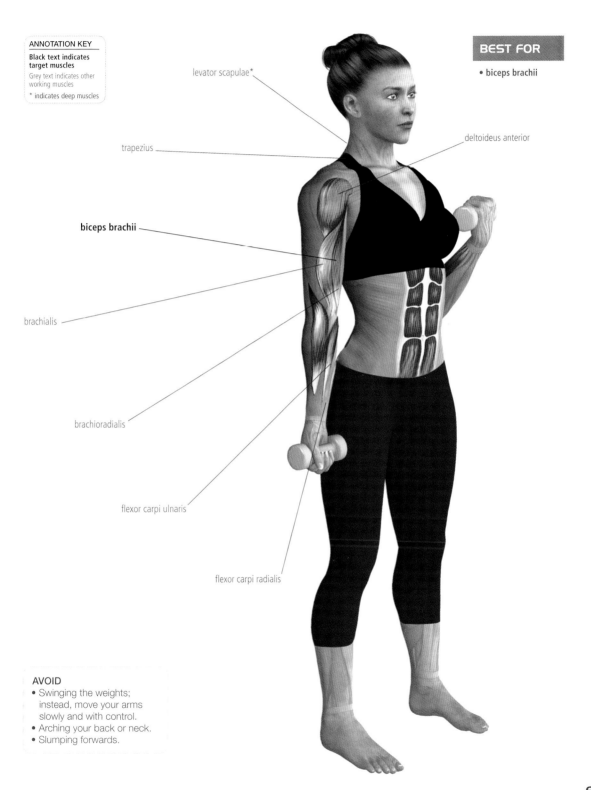

ANNOTATION KEY

Black text indicates
target muscles

Grey text indicates other
working muscles

* indicates deep muscles

levator scapulae*

trapezius

biceps brachii

brachialis

brachioradialis

flexor carpi ulnaris

flexor carpi radialis

deltoideus anterior

BEST FOR

• biceps brachii

AVOID
• Swinging the weights;
  instead, move your arms
  slowly and with control.
• Arching your back or neck.
• Slumping forwards.

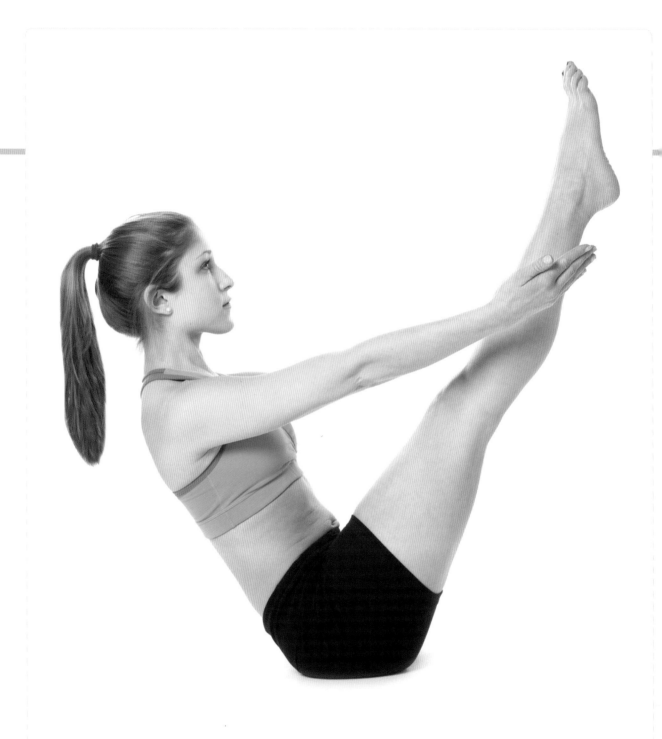

CORE-TRAINING EXERCISES

A sleek, toned midsection and a strong and stable core don't just make you look and feel fitter, they are (quite literally) central to how you function. All of your body's movements, in every conceivable direction, originate in the core, and when you strengthen it, you guard against injury, improve functionality and posture, and build fitness from the inside out. The core is the powerhouse of the body, working so that you can lift, bend and carry all of your daily burdens, from kids to shopping bags. The following exercises train the major core muscles, including the abdominals, the obliques and the muscles that support the spine.

CRUNCH

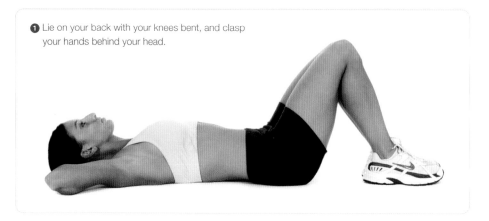

❶ Lie on your back with your knees bent, and clasp your hands behind your head.

❷ Keeping your elbows wide, engage your abdominals, and lift your upper torso to achieve a crunching movement.

❸ Slowly return to the starting position. Repeat 15 times for two sets.

TARGETS
• Abdominals

LEVEL
• Beginner

BENEFITS
• Strengthens the torso
• Improves pelvic and core stability

NOT ADVISABLE IF YOU HAVE . . .
• Back pain
• Neck pain

MODIFICATION
Harder: Lie on your back with your legs outstretched, and your arms over your head. Without lifting your legs, lift your arms and torso in a controlled movement. Continue to curl forwards and grasp your feet.

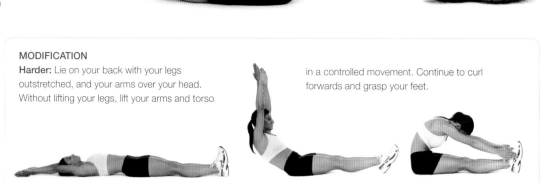

DO IT RIGHT
- Use your shoulders and abdominals to initiate the movement.
- Keep your pelvis in neutral position during the crunching motion.
- Slightly tuck your chin, directing your gaze towards the inner thighs.

AVOID
- Pulling from the neck.
- Tilting your hips towards the floor.

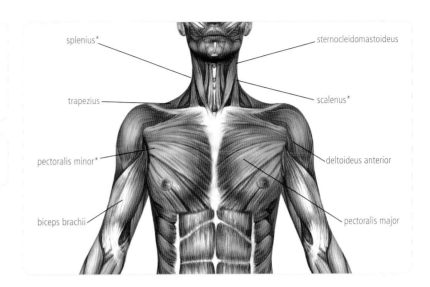

splenius*
sternocleidomastoideus
trapezius
scalenus*
pectoralis minor*
deltoideus anterior
biceps brachii
pectoralis major

ANNOTATION KEY
Black text indicates target muscles
Grey text indicates other working muscles
* indicates deep muscles

BEST FOR
- rectus abdominis
- obliquus internus
- obliquus externus
- transversus abdominis

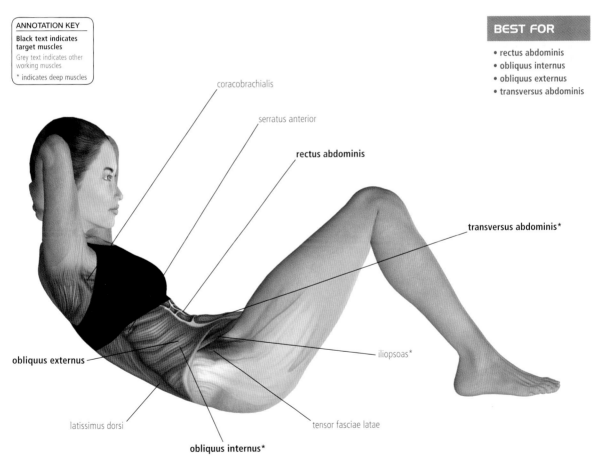

coracobrachialis
serratus anterior
rectus abdominis
transversus abdominis*
obliquus externus
iliopsoas*
latissimus dorsi
tensor fasciae latae
obliquus internus*

HALF CURL

① Lie on your back with your knees bent and arms straight by your sides. Squeeze your legs together and keep your feet flat on the floor.

AVOID
- Curling your neck too far forwards.
- Allowing your feet to raise off the floor.
- Raising up too far.

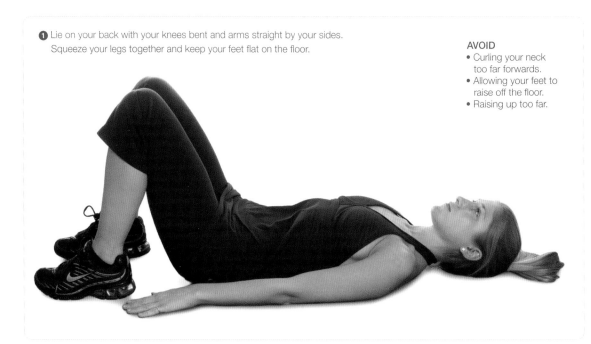

TARGETS
- Upper abdominals

LEVEL
- Beginner

BENEFITS
- Strengthens core muscles
- Increases abdominal endurance

NOT ADVISABLE IF YOU HAVE . . .
- Neck issues

② Using your upper abdominals, curl your upper back and shoulders upwards. Keep your arms parallel to the floor and your lower back flat.

③ Hold for 10 seconds. Return to the starting position, and repeat 10 times.

DO IT RIGHT
- Keep your arms parallel to the floor.

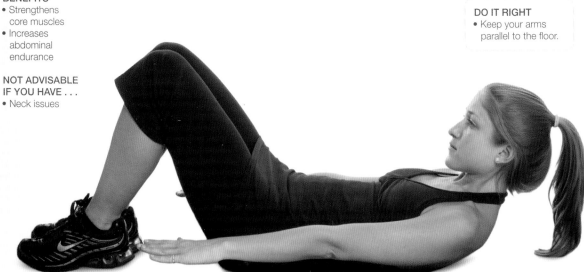

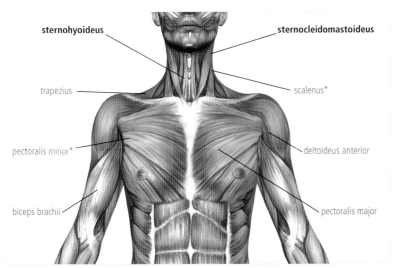

sternohyoideus

sternocleidomastoideus

trapezius

scalenus*

pectoralis minor*

deltoideus anterior

biceps brachii

pectoralis major

BEST FOR

- rectus abdominis
- latissimus dorsi
- pectoralis major
- sternohyoideus
- sternocleidomastoideus
- deltoideus medialis
- biceps brachii
- triceps brachii

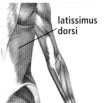

latissimus dorsi

ANNOTATION KEY

Black text indicates target muscles

Grey text indicates other working muscles

* indicates deep muscles

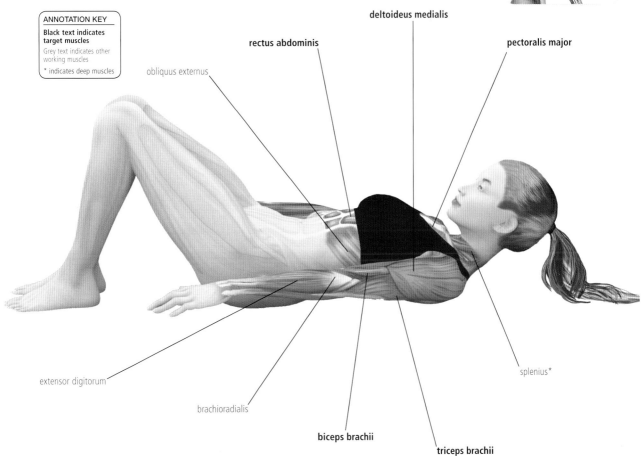

deltoideus medialis

rectus abdominis

pectoralis major

obliquus externus

splenius*

extensor digitorum

brachioradialis

biceps brachii

triceps brachii

SEATED RUSSIAN TWIST

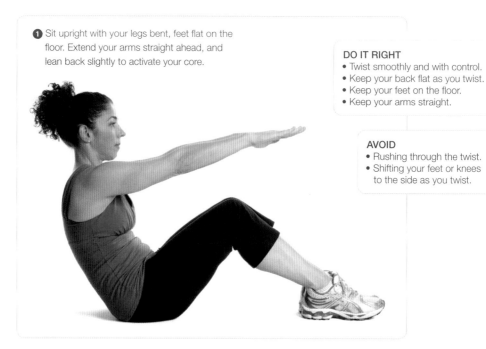

1 Sit upright with your legs bent, feet flat on the floor. Extend your arms straight ahead, and lean back slightly to activate your core.

DO IT RIGHT
- Twist smoothly and with control.
- Keep your back flat as you twist.
- Keep your feet on the floor.
- Keep your arms straight.

AVOID
- Rushing through the twist.
- Shifting your feet or knees to the side as you twist.

TARGETS
- Back
- Obliques
- Upper abdominals

LEVEL
- Intermediate

BENEFITS
- Stabilises and strengthens core

NOT ADVISABLE IF YOU HAVE . . .
- Lower-back pain

2 In a smooth motion, rotate your upper body to the side, and then return to centre. Repeat rotation on the other side.

3 Return to centre, and repeat the full twist, performing three sets of 20.

BEST FOR
- rectus abdominis
- obliquus externus
- obliquus internus
- erector spinae
- transversus abdominis

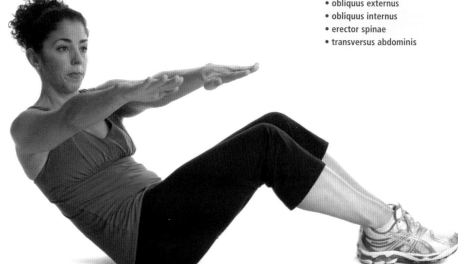

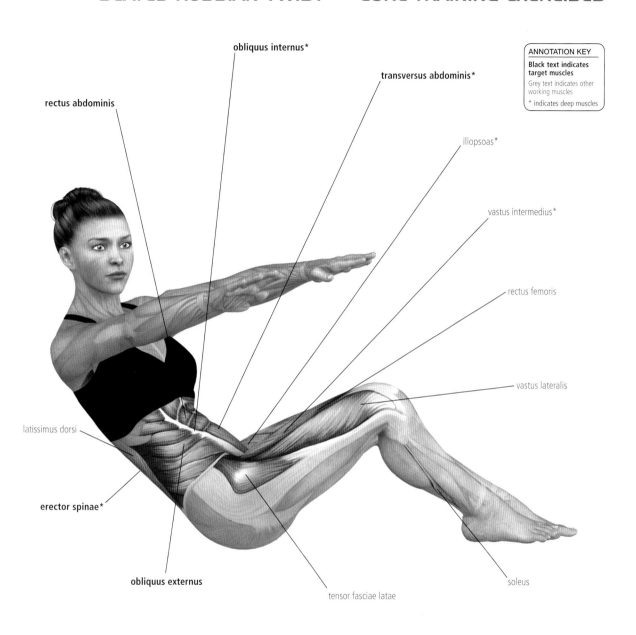

obliquus internus*

transversus abdominis*

ANNOTATION KEY

Black text indicates target muscles

Grey text indicates other working muscles

* indicates deep muscles

rectus abdominis

iliopsoas*

vastus intermedius*

rectus femoris

vastus lateralis

latissimus dorsi

erector spinae*

obliquus externus

tensor fasciae latae

soleus

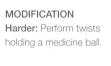

MODIFICATION

Harder: Perform twists holding a medicine ball.

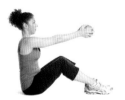

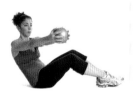

SPINE TWIST

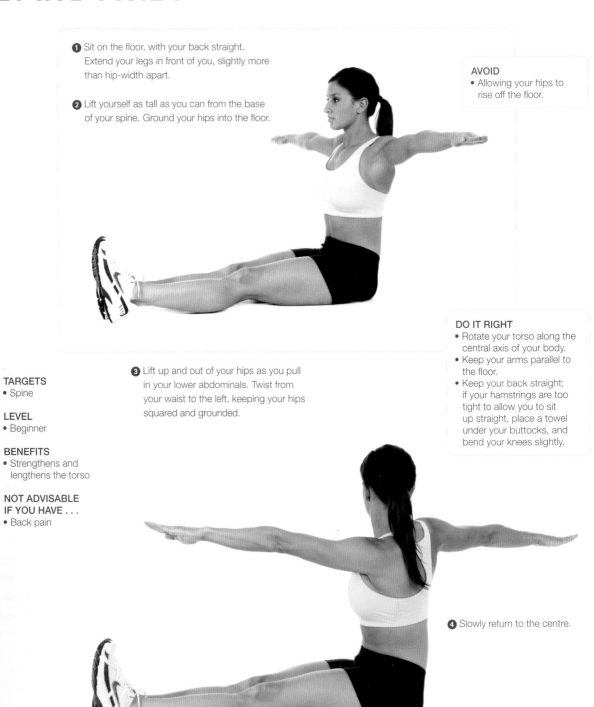

❶ Sit on the floor, with your back straight. Extend your legs in front of you, slightly more than hip-width apart.

❷ Lift yourself as tall as you can from the base of your spine. Ground your hips into the floor.

AVOID
• Allowing your hips to rise off the floor.

❸ Lift up and out of your hips as you pull in your lower abdominals. Twist from your waist to the left, keeping your hips squared and grounded.

DO IT RIGHT
• Rotate your torso along the central axis of your body.
• Keep your arms parallel to the floor.
• Keep your back straight; if your hamstrings are too tight to allow you to sit up straight, place a towel under your buttocks, and bend your knees slightly.

TARGETS
• Spine

LEVEL
• Beginner

BENEFITS
• Strengthens and lengthens the torso

NOT ADVISABLE IF YOU HAVE . . .
• Back pain

❹ Slowly return to the centre.

⑤ Lift up and out of your hips again, twisting in the other direction.

⑥ Return to the centre. Repeat three times in each direction.

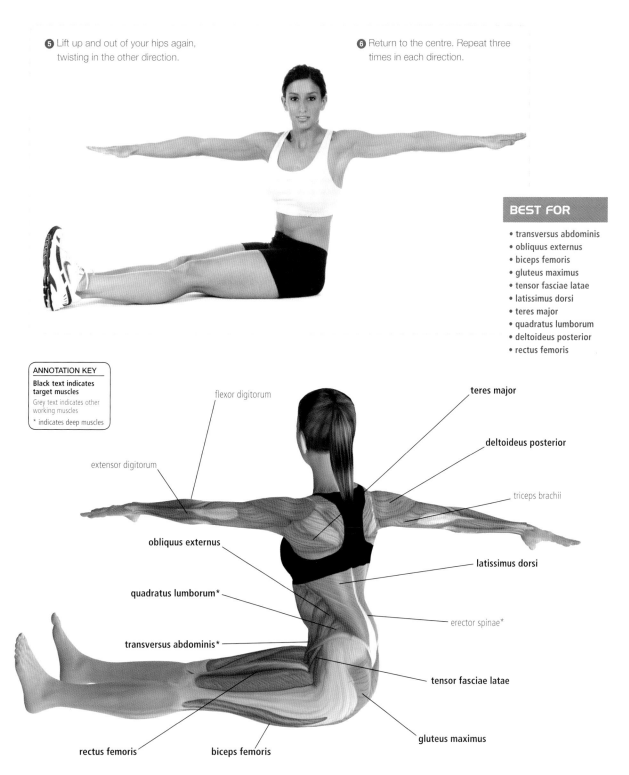

BEST FOR

- transversus abdominis
- obliquus externus
- biceps femoris
- gluteus maximus
- tensor fasciae latae
- latissimus dorsi
- teres major
- quadratus lumborum
- deltoideus posterior
- rectus femoris

ANNOTATION KEY

Black text indicates target muscles

Grey text indicates other working muscles

* indicates deep muscles

flexor digitorum

extensor digitorum

teres major

deltoideus posterior

triceps brachii

obliquus externus

latissimus dorsi

quadratus lumborum*

erector spinae*

transversus abdominis*

tensor fasciae latae

gluteus maximus

rectus femoris

biceps femoris

OBLIQUE ROLL-DOWN

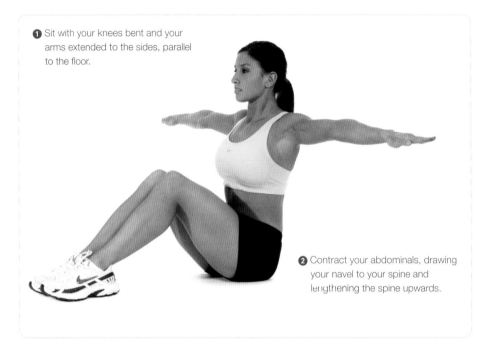

① Sit with your knees bent and your arms extended to the sides, parallel to the floor.

② Contract your abdominals, drawing your navel to your spine and lengthening the spine upwards.

TARGETS
• Obliques

LEVEL
• Advanced

BENEFITS
• Tightens the obliques and abdominals

NOT ADVISABLE IF YOU HAVE . . .
• Herniated disc

③ Roll backwards while simultaneously rotating your torso to one side.

④ Maintaining spinal flexion, rotate your torso back to the centre.

AVOID
• Tensing your neck and shoulder muscles.

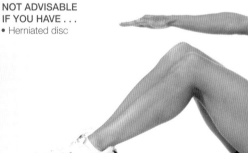

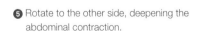

⑤ Rotate to the other side, deepening the abdominal contraction.

⑥ Return back to the centre, and repeat sequence four to six times on each side.

DO IT RIGHT

- Lengthen your arms as you roll down to create opposition throughout the torso.
- Relax and lengthen your neck to prevent straining.
- Articulate your spine while rolling up and down.

ANNOTATION KEY

Black text indicates target muscles

Grey text indicates other working muscles

* indicates deep muscles

deltoideus posterior

teres major

triceps brachii

latissimus dorsi

gluteus medius*

BEST FOR

- obliquus externus
- obliquus internus
- rectus abdominis
- transversus abdominis

rectus abdominis

transversus abdominis*

obliquus internus*

biceps brachii

brachioradialis

rectus femoris

extensor digitorum

biceps femoris

obliquus externus

sartorius

tensor fasciae latae

BICYCLE CRUNCH

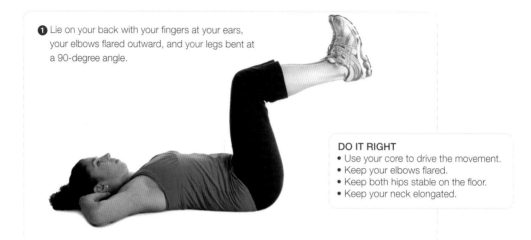

❶ Lie on your back with your fingers at your ears, your elbows flared outward, and your legs bent at a 90-degree angle.

DO IT RIGHT
• Use your core to drive the movement.
• Keep your elbows flared.
• Keep both hips stable on the floor.
• Keep your neck elongated.

❷ Roll up with your torso, reaching one elbow diagonally towards the opposite knee. At the same time, extend the other leg forwards.

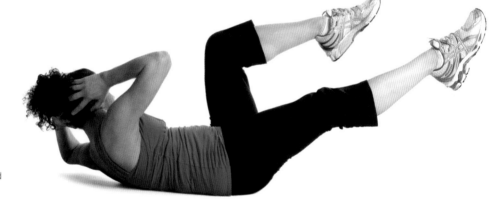

TARGETS
• Obliques
• Upper abdominals

LEVEL
• Intermediate

BENEFITS
• Stabilises core
• Strengthens and tones obliques and upper abdominals
• Hip flexors

NOT ADVISABLE IF YOU HAVE . . .
• Neck issues
• Lower-back pain

❸ Release, and repeat on the other side. Continue to alternate, completing 15 crunches in each direction.

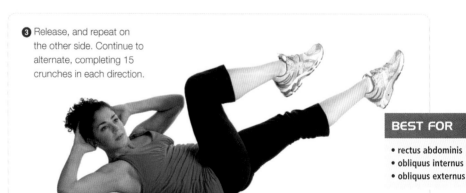

BEST FOR
• rectus abdominis
• obliquus internus
• obliquus externus

MODIFICATION

Similar level of difficulty:
Keep both feet flexed
throughout the exercise.

AVOID
• Arching your back or raising
  your lower back off the floor.
• Pulling your head upwards
  with your hands.

ANNOTATION KEY

**Black text indicates
target muscles**

Grey text indicates other
working muscles

* indicates deep muscles

iliopsoas*

tensor fasciae latae

sartorius

rectus femoris

intercostales interni*

tibialis anterior

intercostales externi

rectus abdominis

obliquus internus*

obliquus externus

MODIFICATION

Easier: Begin with one foot
on the floor, and place the
outside of your other foot on
top of your thigh near your
knee. As you crunch, bring
your opposite elbow

towards that top knee.
Complete five reps on
one side, then switch
sides and repeat.

THE BOAT

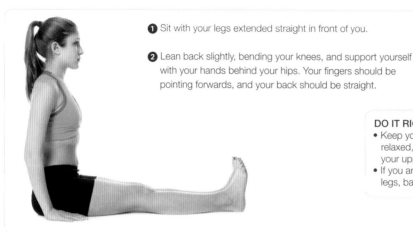

❶ Sit with your legs extended straight in front of you.

❷ Lean back slightly, bending your knees, and support yourself with your hands behind your hips. Your fingers should be pointing forwards, and your back should be straight.

DO IT RIGHT
- Keep your neck elongated and relaxed, minimising the tension in your upper spine.
- If you are unable to straighten your legs, balance with your knees bent.

❸ Exhale, and lift your feet off the floor as you lean back from your shoulders. Find your balance point between your sit bones and your tailbone.

❹ Slowly straighten your legs in front of you so that they form a 45-degree angle with your torso. Point your toes. Lift your arms to your sides, parallel to the floor.

❺ Pull your abdominals in towards your spine as they work to keep your balance. Stretch your arms forwards through your fingertips, and elongate the back of your neck.

❻ Hold for 10 to 20 seconds.

TARGETS
- Abdominals
- Hip flexors

LEVEL
- Advanced

BENEFITS
- Strengthens abdominals, hip flexors, spine and thighs
- Stretches hamstrings

NOT ADVISABLE IF YOU HAVE . . .
- Neck injury
- Headache
- Lower-back pain

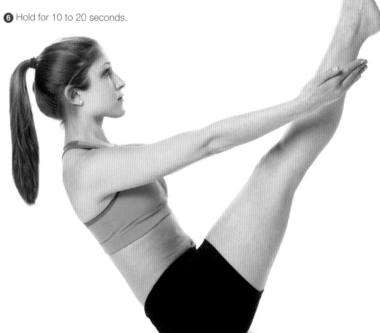

BEST FOR

- rectus abdominis
- obliquus internus
- obliquus externus
- iliopsoas
- transversus abdominis
- vastus intermedius
- rectus femoris
- erector spinae

AVOID
- Rounding your spine, which places pressure on your lower back.

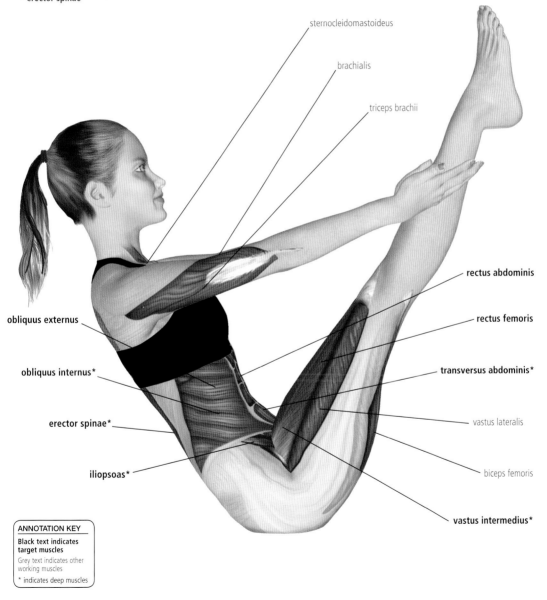

sternocleidomastoideus

brachialis

triceps brachii

rectus abdominis

rectus femoris

transversus abdominis*

vastus lateralis

biceps femoris

vastus intermedius*

obliquus externus

obliquus internus*

erector spinae*

iliopsoas*

ANNOTATION KEY

Black text indicates target muscles

Grey text indicates other working muscles

* indicates deep muscles

85

V-UP

❶ Lie on your back with your legs raised a few inches from the floor.

❷ Inhale, reaching your arms towards the ceiling as you lift your head and shoulders off the floor.

AVOID
• Using momentum to carry you through the exercise; instead, use your abdominal muscles to lift your legs and torso.

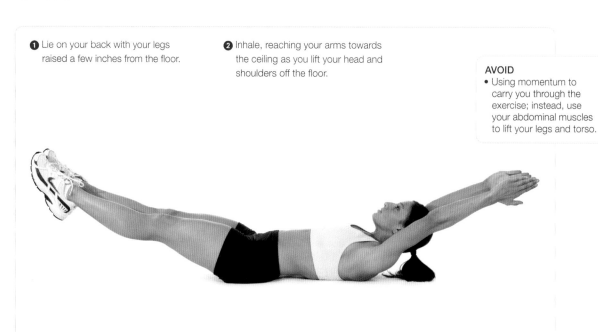

TARGETS
• Abdominals

LEVEL
• Advanced

BENEFITS
• Strengthens the abdominals
• Increases spinal flexibility

NOT ADVISABLE IF YOU HAVE . . .
• Advanced osteoporosis
• Herniated disc

❸ Exhale, and keeping them straight, begin lifting your legs to a 45-degree angle from the floor.

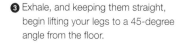

DO IT RIGHT
• Articulate through the spine on the way up and on the way down.
• Keep your neck elongated and relaxed, minimising the tension in your upper spine.

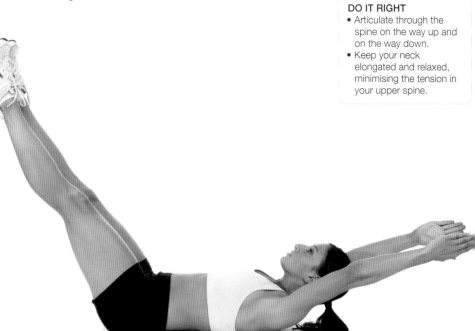

4 While rolling through the spine, lift your rib cage off the floor to just before the sit bones.

5 Inhale, and reach your arms towards your toes while maintaining a C curve in your back. Exhale, and roll down the spine by articulating one vertebra at a time. Return to the starting position.

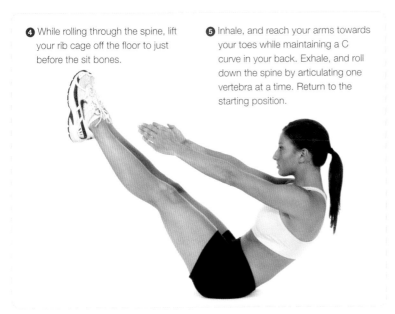

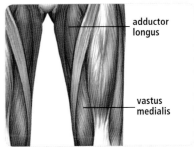

adductor longus

vastus medialis

BEST FOR

- rectus abdominis
- tensor fasciae latae
- rectus femoris
- vastus lateralis
- vastus medialis
- vastus intermedius
- adductor longus
- pectineus
- brachialis

ANNOTATION KEY

Black text indicates target muscles
Grey text indicates other working muscles
* indicates deep muscles

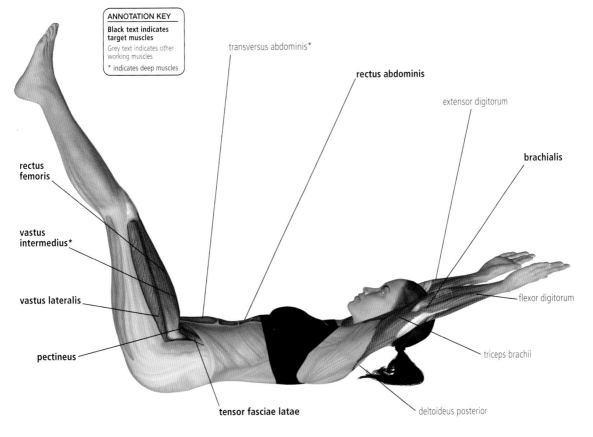

transversus abdominis*

rectus abdominis

extensor digitorum

brachialis

rectus femoris

vastus intermedius*

vastus lateralis

flexor digitorum

pectineus

triceps brachii

tensor fasciae latae

deltoideus posterior

BACKWARDS BALL STRETCH

DO IT RIGHT
- Maintain good balance throughout the stretch.
- Move slowly and in a controlled manner.
- Keep your head on the ball until you have dropped your knees all the way down as you release from the stretch.

AVOID
- Allowing the ball to shift to the side.
- Holding the extended position for too long, or until you feel dizzy.

TARGETS
- Thoracic and upper-lumbar spine
- Abdominals

LEVEL
- Advanced

BENEFITS
- Stretches thoracic spine
- Increases spinal extension
- Stretches abdominals and large back muscles

NOT ADVISABLE IF YOU HAVE . . .
- Lower-back pain
- Balancing difficulty

1 Sit on a Swiss ball in a well-balanced, neutral position, with your hips directly over the centre of the ball.

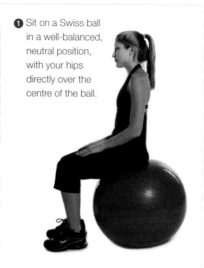

2 Raise your arms while maintaining good balance, and begin to extend them behind you.

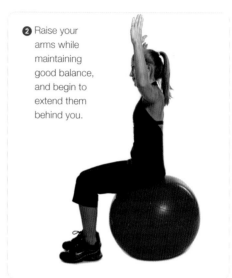

3 As you continue to extend your hands backwards, walk your feet forwards, allowing the ball to roll up your spine.

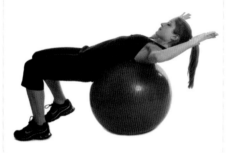

4 As your hands touch the floor, extend your legs as far forwards as you comfortably can. Hold this position for 10 seconds.

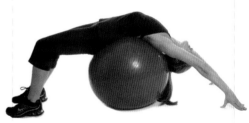

5 To deepen the stretch, extend your arms, and walk your legs and hands closer to the ball. Hold this position for 10 seconds.

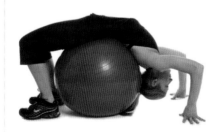

6 To release the stretch, bend your knees, drop your hips to the floor, lift your head off the ball, and then walk back to the starting position.

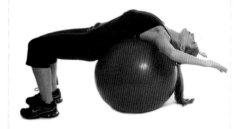

MODIFICATION

Easier: Follow steps 1 through 3, but rather than extend your hands to the floor, clasp them behind your head. Hold this position for 10 seconds, and release.

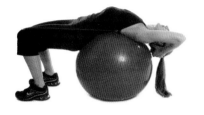

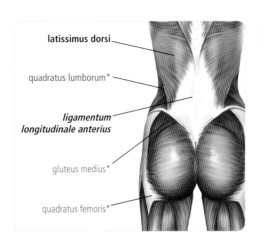

latissimus dorsi

quadratus lumborum*

ligamentum longitudinale anterius

gluteus medius*

quadratus femoris*

BEST FOR

- deltoideus medialis
- iliopsoas
- latissimus dorsi
- serratus anterior
- pectoralis major
- pectoralis minor
- ligamentum longitudinale anterius

ANNOTATION KEY

Black text indicates target muscles
Grey text indicates other working muscles
Black italics indicates ligaments
* indicates deep muscles

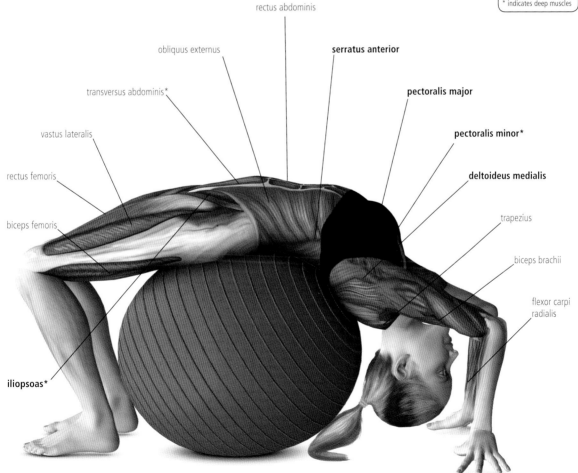

rectus abdominis

obliquus externus

transversus abdominis*

vastus lateralis

rectus femoris

biceps femoris

iliopsoas*

serratus anterior

pectoralis major

pectoralis minor*

deltoideus medialis

trapezius

biceps brachii

flexor carpi radialis

PLANK

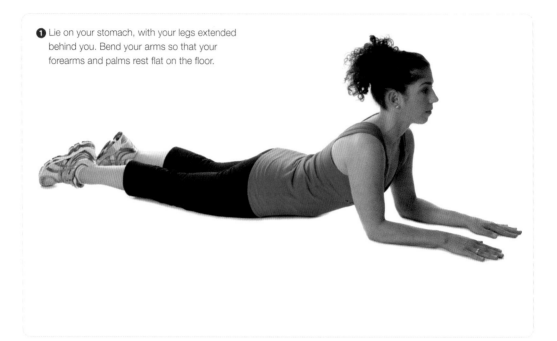

① Lie on your stomach, with your legs extended behind you. Bend your arms so that your forearms and palms rest flat on the floor.

TARGETS
• Abdominals
• Back
• Obliques

LEVEL
• Beginner

BENEFITS
• Strengthens and stabilises core

NOT ADVISABLE IF YOU HAVE . . .
• Shoulder injury
• Severe back pain

② Bend your knees, supporting your weight between your knees and your forearms, and then push through with your forearms to bring your shoulders up towards the ceiling as you straighten your legs.

③ With control, lower your shoulders until you feel them coming together at your back. Hold for 30 seconds, building up to 2 minutes if desired.

BEST FOR
• erector spinae
• transversus abdominis
• rectus abdominis
• obliquus externus
• obliquus internus

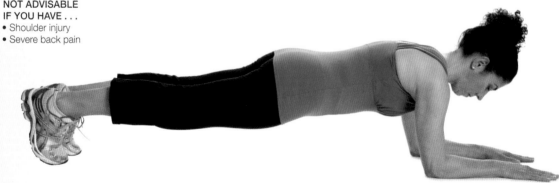

AVOID
- Allowing your shoulders to collapse into your shoulder joints.
- Arching your neck.
- Allowing your back to sag.

DO IT RIGHT
- Keep your abs tight.
- Keep your body in a straight line.
- Lengthen through your neck.
- Start by holding for just 15 seconds, if desired.

ANNOTATION KEY
Black text indicates target muscles
Grey text indicates other working muscles
* indicates deep muscles

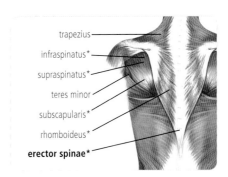

trapezius
infraspinatus*
supraspinatus*
teres minor
subscapularis*
rhomboideus*
erector spinae*

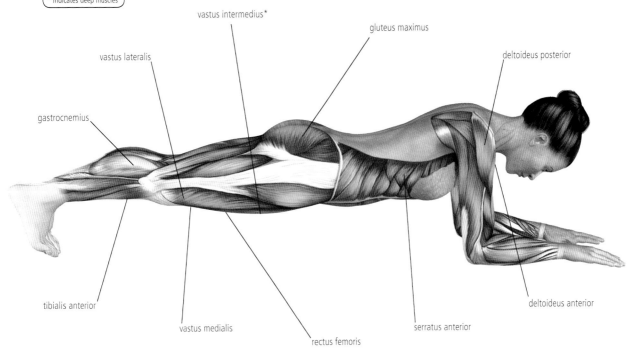

vastus intermedius*
gluteus maximus
deltoideus posterior
vastus lateralis
gastrocnemius
deltoideus anterior
tibialis anterior
vastus medialis
rectus femoris
serratus anterior

MODIFICATION
Harder: While in the plank position, lift and lower your legs one at a time. Keep the rest of your body still, and your abs engaged throughout.

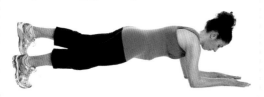

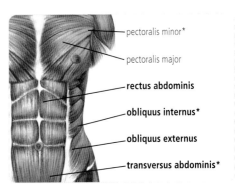

pectoralis minor*
pectoralis major
rectus abdominis
obliquus internus*
obliquus externus
transversus abdominis*

SWISS BALL TRANSVERSE ABS

1 Position yourself on your toes with your arms bent and forearms resting on top of a Swiss ball.

2 Form a long, straight line from your ankles to your shoulders.

3 Hold this position for as long as you can.

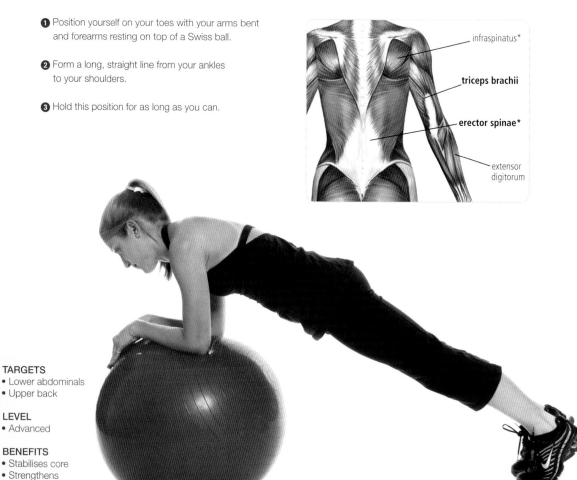

infraspinatus*

triceps brachii

erector spinae*

extensor digitorum

TARGETS
• Lower abdominals
• Upper back

LEVEL
• Advanced

BENEFITS
• Stabilises core
• Strengthens abdominals
• Strengthens lower back

NOT ADVISABLE IF YOU HAVE . . .
• Neck pain
• Lower-back pain

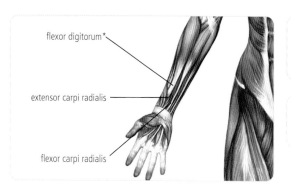

flexor digitorum*

extensor carpi radialis

flexor carpi radialis

DO IT RIGHT
• Breathe easily and normally.
• Activate your abs so that you maintain neutral alignment.

AVOID
• Allowing your lower back to drop out of alignment.

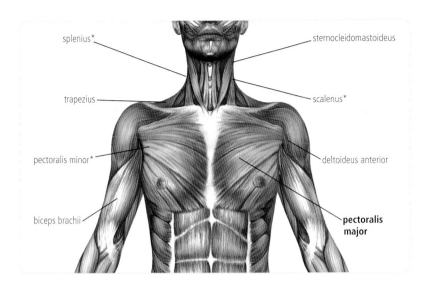

splenius*

sternocleidomastoideus

trapezius

scalenus*

pectoralis minor*

deltoideus anterior

biceps brachii

pectoralis major

BEST FOR

- rectus abdominis
- transversus abdominis
- rectus femoris
- iliopsoas
- latissimus dorsi
- obliquus externus
- obliquus internus
- pectoralis major
- teres major
- triceps brachii
- erector spinae

ANNOTATION KEY

Black text indicates target muscles

Grey text indicates other working muscles

* indicates deep muscles

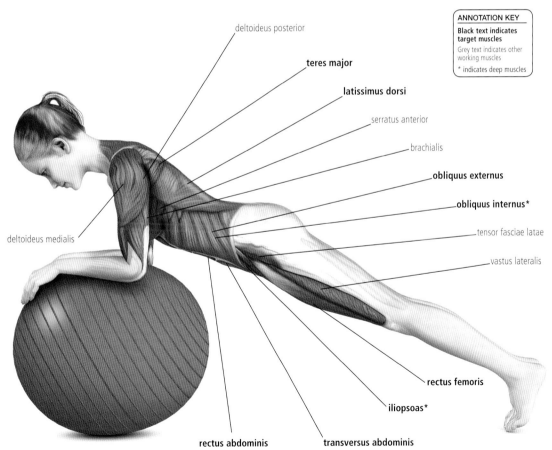

deltoideus posterior

teres major

latissimus dorsi

serratus anterior

brachialis

obliquus externus

obliquus internus*

tensor fasciae latae

vastus lateralis

deltoideus medialis

rectus femoris

iliopsoas*

rectus abdominis

transversus abdominis

SWISS BALL ROLLOUT

BEST FOR

- **rectus abdominis**
- **erector spinae**

❶ Kneel in front of a Swiss ball, with your hands resting on the ball.

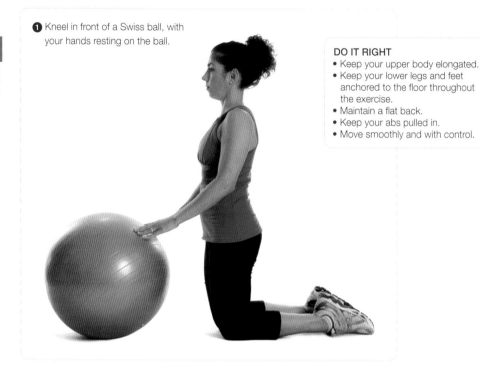

DO IT RIGHT
- Keep your upper body elongated.
- Keep your lower legs and feet anchored to the floor throughout the exercise.
- Maintain a flat back.
- Keep your abs pulled in.
- Move smoothly and with control.

TARGETS
- Back
- Upper abdominals

LEVEL
- Intermediate

BENEFITS
- Stabilises core

NOT ADVISABLE IF YOU HAVE . . .
- Lower-back issues
- Knee issues

❷ Use your hands to roll the ball slightly in front of you as you begin to lean forwards.

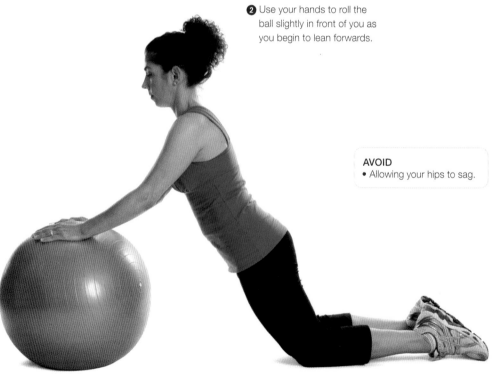

AVOID
- Allowing your hips to sag.

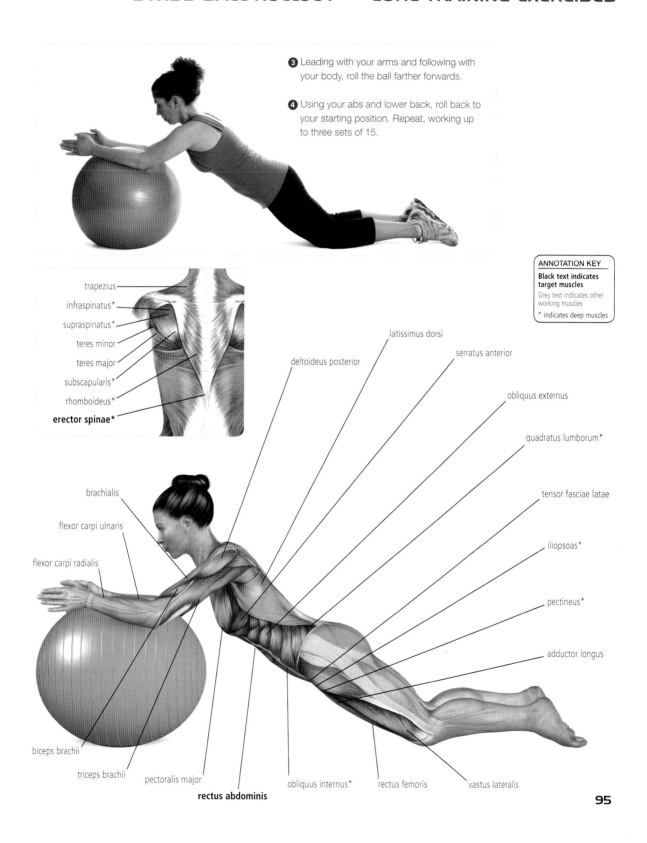

3 Leading with your arms and following with your body, roll the ball farther forwards.

4 Using your abs and lower back, roll back to your starting position. Repeat, working up to three sets of 15.

ANNOTATION KEY

Black text indicates target muscles

Grey text indicates other working muscles

* indicates deep muscles

trapezius

infraspinatus*

supraspinatus*

teres minor

teres major

subscapularis*

rhomboideus*

erector spinae*

latissimus dorsi

deltoideus posterior

serratus anterior

obliquus externus

quadratus lumborum*

brachialis

flexor carpi ulnaris

flexor carpi radialis

tensor fasciae latae

iliopsoas*

pectineus*

adductor longus

biceps brachii

triceps brachii

pectoralis major

rectus abdominis

obliquus internus*

rectus femoris

vastus lateralis

FOAM ROLLER CALF PRESS

DO IT RIGHT
- Form a long, straight line with your lifted leg.
- Keep your hips elevated throughout the exercise.

AVOID
- Allowing your shoulders to lift towards your ears.
- Bending your knees.
- Bending your elbows.

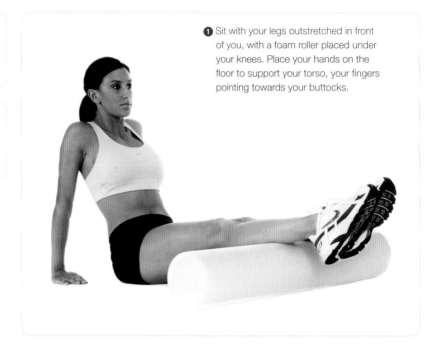

1 Sit with your legs outstretched in front of you, with a foam roller placed under your knees. Place your hands on the floor to support your torso, your fingers pointing towards your buttocks.

TARGETS
- Abdominals
- Upper arms
- Shoulder stabilisers
- Hamstrings

LEVEL
- Advanced

BENEFITS
- Improves core, pelvic and shoulder stability

NOT ADVISABLE IF YOU HAVE . . .
- Wrist pain
- Shoulder pain
- Knee issues

2 Press into the floor to lift your hips, keeping your legs firm.

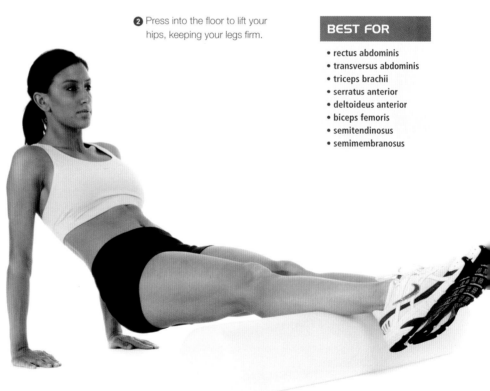

BEST FOR
- **rectus abdominis**
- **transversus abdominis**
- **triceps brachii**
- **serratus anterior**
- **deltoideus anterior**
- **biceps femoris**
- **semitendinosus**
- **semimembranosus**

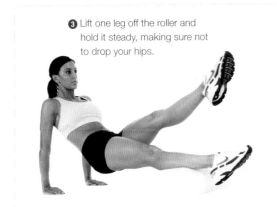

3 Lift one leg off the roller and hold it steady, making sure not to drop your hips.

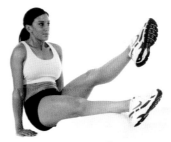

4 Keep your leg lifted, and press your opposite leg into the roller, drawing your hips back towards your hands.

5 Return to the starting position, rolling your calf muscle along the roller and keeping your lifted leg straight in the air. Repeat 15 times on each leg.

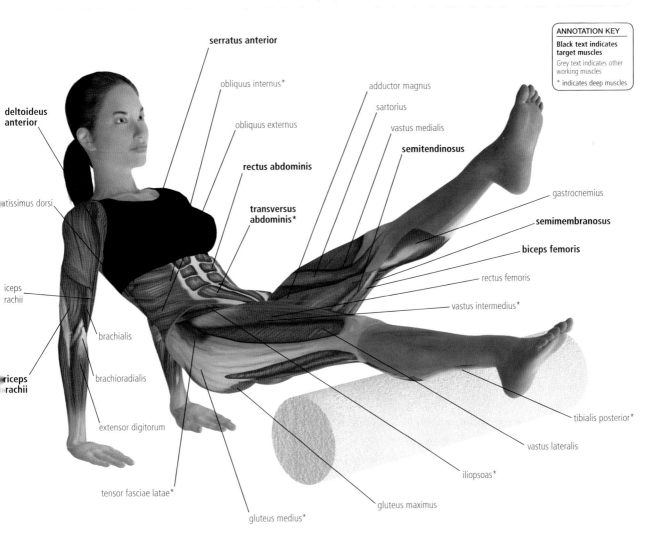

ANNOTATION KEY

Black text indicates target muscles

Grey text indicates other working muscles

* indicates deep muscles

serratus anterior

obliquus internus*

obliquus externus

rectus abdominis

transversus abdominis*

adductor magnus

sartorius

vastus medialis

semitendinosus

gastrocnemius

semimembranosus

biceps femoris

rectus femoris

vastus intermedius*

tibialis posterior*

vastus lateralis

iliopsoas*

gluteus maximus

gluteus medius*

tensor fasciae latae*

extensor digitorum

brachioradialis

brachialis

deltoideus anterior

tissimus dorsi

iceps rachii

riceps rachii

97

FOAM ROLLER DIAGONAL CRUNCH

❶ Lie lengthwise on a foam roller so that it follows the line of your spine. Your buttocks and shoulders should both be in contact with the roller.

❷ With your legs straight and your feet pressed firmly into the floor, extend your arms over your head.

DO IT RIGHT
- Keep your legs firm throughout exercise.
- Keep your buttocks and shoulders in contact with the roller throughout exercise.

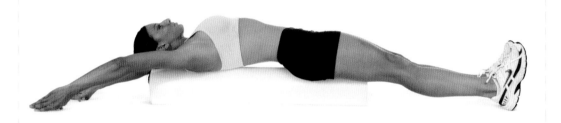

❸ Raise your head, neck, and shoulders as if to do a crunch. Leave your left leg and right arm down on the floor, using your hand for support. Raise your right leg and right arm, and reach for your ankle.

TARGETS
- Upper arms
- Shoulder stabilisers
- Abdominals
- Hamstrings

LEVEL
- Advanced

BENEFITS
- Improves core, pelvic and shoulder stability

NOT ADVISABLE IF YOU HAVE . . .
- Back pain
- Neck pain

❹ Slowly roll down the roller, dropping your raised arm and leg. Repeat on the opposite leg and arm. Repeat 15 times on each side.

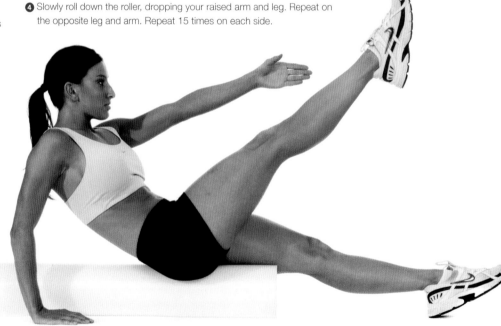

MODIFICATION

Harder: Keep one leg on the floor for support, and reach both arms towards the raised leg as you crunch up.

ANNOTATION KEY

Black text indicates target muscles

Grey text indicates other working muscles

* indicates deep muscles

AVOID

- Allowing your shoulders to lift towards your ears.
- Bending your knees.

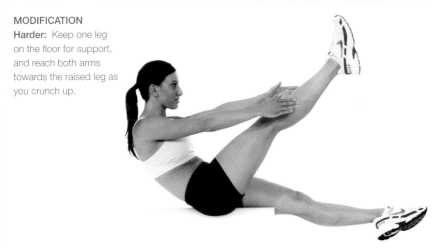

pectoralis major

coracobrachialis*

biceps brachii

serratus anterior

rectus abdominis

obliquus internus*

obliquus externus

pectoralis minor*

rectus femoris

transversus abdominis*

vastus lateralis

trapezius

semimembranosus

semitendinosus

vastus intermedius*

triceps brachii

biceps femoris

sartorius

deltoideus anterior

vastus medialis

iliopsoas*

gluteus maximus

tensor fasciae latae*

FOAM ROLLER SUPINE MARCHES

❶ Lie lengthwise on a foam roller so that it follows the line of your spine. Place your arms on the floor by your sides, bending your knees so that your feet rest flat on the floor.

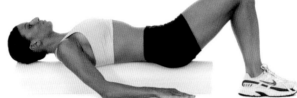

BEST FOR

- rectus abdominis
- transversus abdominis
- obliquus internus
- obliquus externus
- iliopsoas
- sartorius
- biceps femoris
- rectus femoris

❷ Pointing your toes and keeping your hips from lifting or shifting, raise one knee towards your chest.

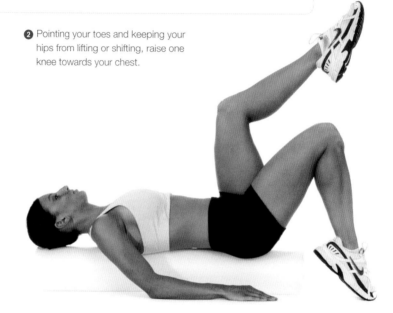

TARGETS
- Abdominals
- Upper arms
- Hip flexors
- Quadriceps

LEVEL
- Advanced

BENEFITS
- Improves core and pelvic stability

NOT ADVISABLE IF YOU HAVE . . .
- Lower-back pain
- Neck pain
- Shoulder pain

❸ Switch legs, again being careful not to allow your hips to lift.

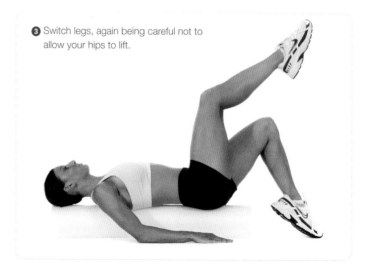

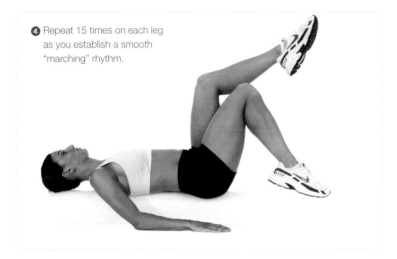

4 Repeat 15 times on each leg as you establish a smooth "marching" rhythm.

AVOID
- Allowing your shoulders to lift towards your ears.
- Allowing your hips and lower back to lift off the roller during the movement.

DO IT RIGHT
- Keep your logs and your toes pointed.
- Relax your neck and shoulders throughout the exercise.
- Keep your hands and forearms flat on the floor.

ANNOTATION KEY

Black text indicates target muscles

Grey text indicates other working muscles

* indicates deep muscles

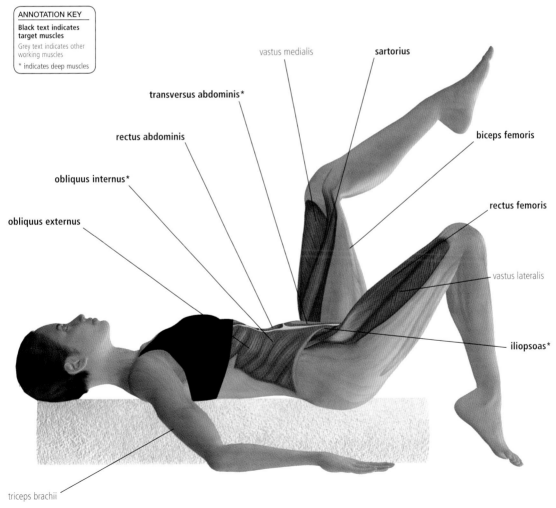

vastus medialis

sartorius

transversus abdominis*

biceps femoris

rectus abdominis

rectus femoris

obliquus internus*

vastus lateralis

obliquus externus

iliopsoas*

triceps brachii

TINY STEPS

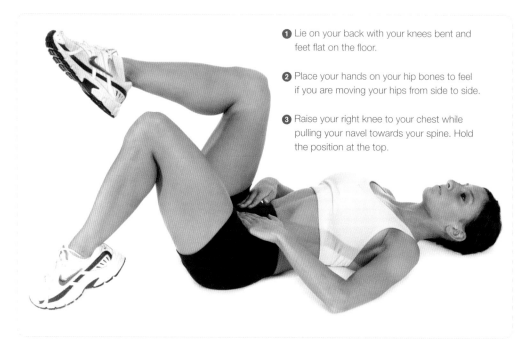

1 Lie on your back with your knees bent and feet flat on the floor.

2 Place your hands on your hip bones to feel if you are moving your hips from side to side.

3 Raise your right knee to your chest while pulling your navel towards your spine. Hold the position at the top.

4 As you continue to pull your navel towards your spine, lower your right leg onto the floor while controlling any movement in your hips.

5 Alternate legs to complete the full movement. Repeat six to eight times.

TARGETS
• Lower abdominals

LEVEL
• Beginner

BENEFITS
• Develops lower-abdominal stability

NOT ADVISABLE IF YOU HAVE . . .
• Sharp lower-back pain that radiates down the legs

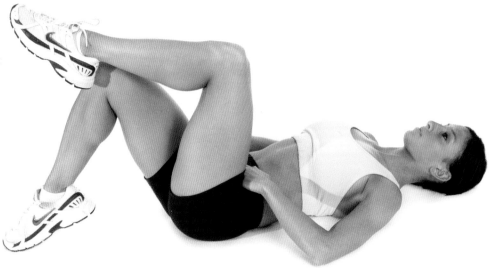

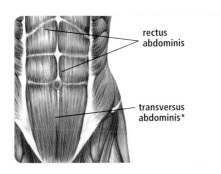

rectus
abdominis

transversus
abdominis*

AVOID
• Allowing your hips to
move back and forth
while legs are mobilised.

DO IT RIGHT
• Pull your navel in towards
your spine throughout the
exercise.

BEST FOR

• rectus abdominis
• rectus femoris
• tensor fasciae latae
• gluteus maximus
• transversus
abdominis
• obliquus internus

ANNOTATION KEY
**Black text indicates
target muscles**
Grey text indicates other
working muscles
* indicates deep muscles

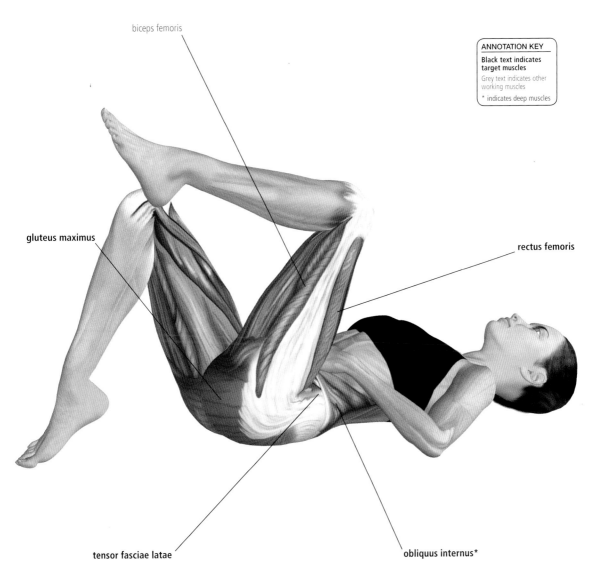

biceps femoris

gluteus maximus

rectus femoris

tensor fasciae latae

obliquus internus*

DOUBLE-LEG ABDOMINAL PRESS

1 Lie on your back with your knees and feet lifted in tabletop position, your thighs making a 90-degree angle with your upper body. Place your hands on the front of your knees, your fingers facing upwards, one palm on each leg.

AVOID
- Holding your breath while performing the exercise.

TARGETS
- Total body

LEVEL
- Intermediate

BENEFITS
- Strengthens core, hip flexors and upper arms

NOT ADVISABLE IF YOU HAVE . . .
- Back pain
- Hip pain

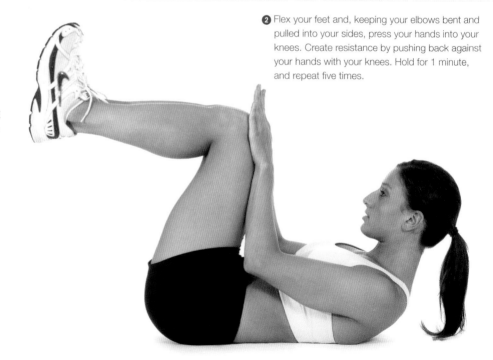

2 Flex your feet and, keeping your elbows bent and pulled into your sides, press your hands into your knees. Create resistance by pushing back against your hands with your knees. Hold for 1 minute, and repeat five times.

104

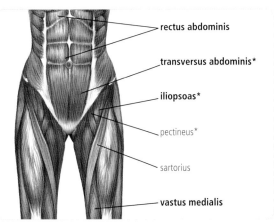

rectus abdominis

transversus abdominis*

iliopsoas*

pectineus*

sartorius

vastus medialis

BEST FOR

- rectus abdominis
- transversus abdominis
- triceps brachii
- iliopsoas
- vastus medialis
- vastus lateralis
- vastus intermedius
- rectus femoris

DO IT RIGHT

- Keep your elbows pulled in towards your sides.
- Relax your shoulders and neck.
- Flex your feet and press your knees together.
- Tuck your tailbone up towards the ceiling.

ANNOTATION KEY

Black text indicates target muscles

Grey text indicates other working muscles

* indicates deep muscles

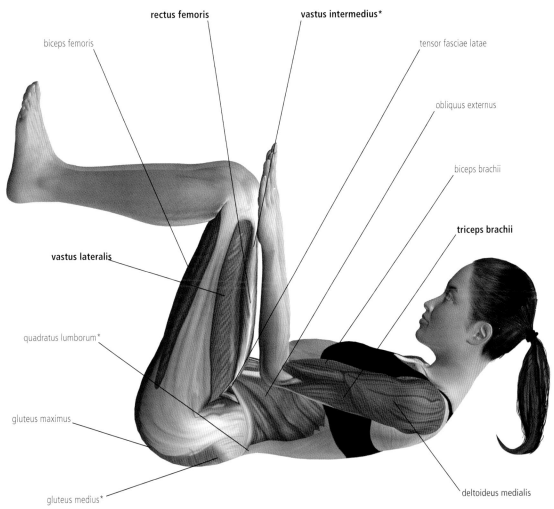

rectus femoris

vastus intermedius*

biceps femoris

tensor fasciae latae

obliquus externus

biceps brachii

triceps brachii

vastus lateralis

quadratus lumborum*

gluteus maximus

gluteus medius*

deltoideus medialis

THE TWIST

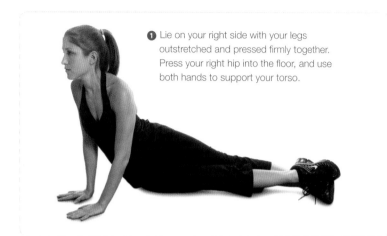

1 Lie on your right side with your legs outstretched and pressed firmly together. Press your right hip into the floor, and use both hands to support your torso.

DO IT RIGHT
- Keep your limbs elongated as much as possible.
- Keep your shoulders stable.
- Lift your hips up high to reduce the weight on your upper body.

TARGETS
- Abdominals
- Shoulders

LEVEL
- Advanced

BENEFITS
- Provides a total-body workout
- Builds endurance

NOT ADVISABLE IF YOU HAVE . . .
- Shoulder issues
- Back pain
- Wrist injury

2 Position your right hand directly beneath your shoulder and press your body upwards until you form a straight line from shoulder to feet.

3 Drawing your navel into your spine, extend your left arm towards the ceiling.

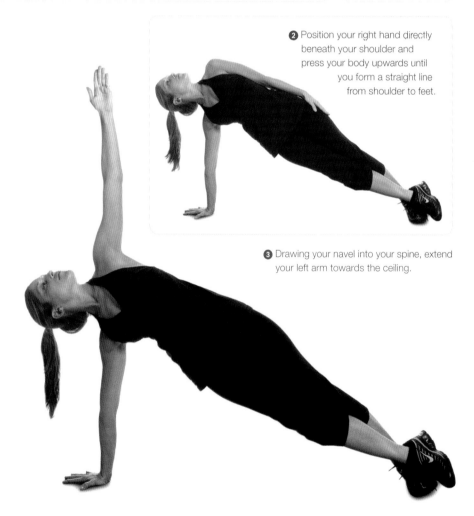

④ Bring your left arm down and across your torso, rotating the upper body to the right. Hold for a count of 10.

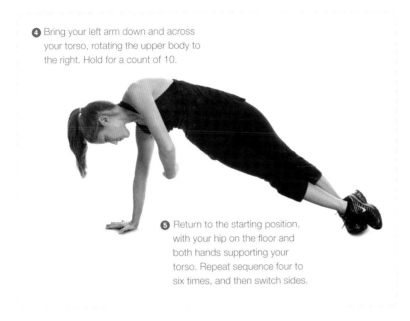

⑤ Return to the starting position, with your hip on the floor and both hands supporting your torso. Repeat sequence four to six times, and then switch sides.

BEST FOR

- latissimus dorsi
- rectus abdominis
- obliquus internus
- obliquus externus
- transversus abdominis
- adductor magnus
- adductor longus
- deltoideus medialis

AVOID
- Allowing your shoulder to sink into its socket.

ANNOTATION KEY
Black text indicates target muscles
Grey text indicates other working muscles
* indicates deep muscles

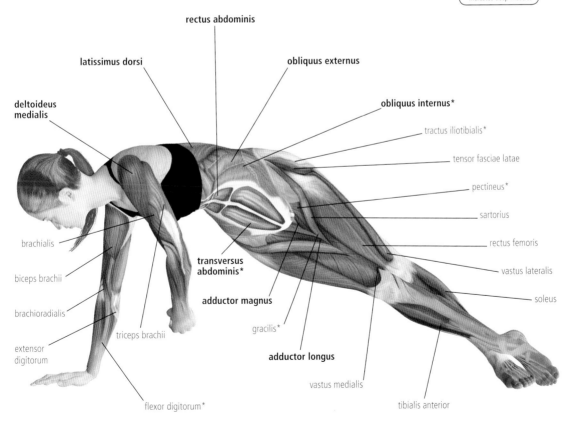

rectus abdominis

latissimus dorsi

obliquus externus

obliquus internus*

deltoideus medialis

tractus iliotibialis*

tensor fasciae latae

pectineus*

sartorius

brachialis

rectus femoris

biceps brachii

transversus abdominis*

vastus lateralis

brachioradialis

adductor magnus

soleus

triceps brachii

gracilis*

extensor digitorum

adductor longus

flexor digitorum*

vastus medialis

tibialis anterior

STANDING KNEE CRUNCH

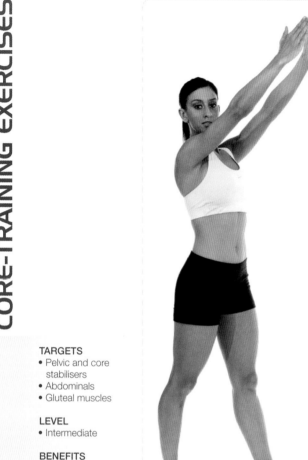

❶ Stand tall with your left leg in front of the right, and extend your hands up towards the ceiling, your arms straight.

BEST FOR

- rectus abdominis
- obliquus internus
- obliquus externus
- transversus abdominis
- gluteus maximus
- gluteus medius
- tensor fasciae latae
- piriformis
- iliopsoas
- gastrocnemius
- soleus

TARGETS
- Pelvic and core stabilisers
- Abdominals
- Gluteal muscles

LEVEL
- Intermediate

BENEFITS
- Strengthens core
- Strengthens calves and gluteal muscles
- Improves balance

NOT ADVISABLE IF YOU HAVE . . .
- Knee pain

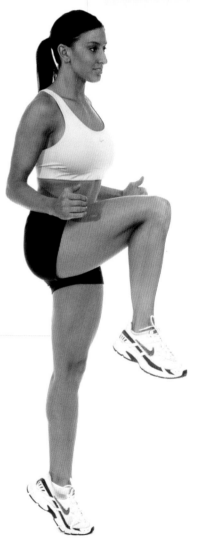

❷ Shift your weight onto your left foot, and raise your right knee to the height of your hips. Simultaneously go up on the toes of your left leg, while pulling your elbows down by your sides, your hands making fists. This creates the crunch.

❸ Pause at the top of the movement, and then return to the starting position. Repeat the sequence with your right leg as the standing leg. Repeat 10 times on each leg.

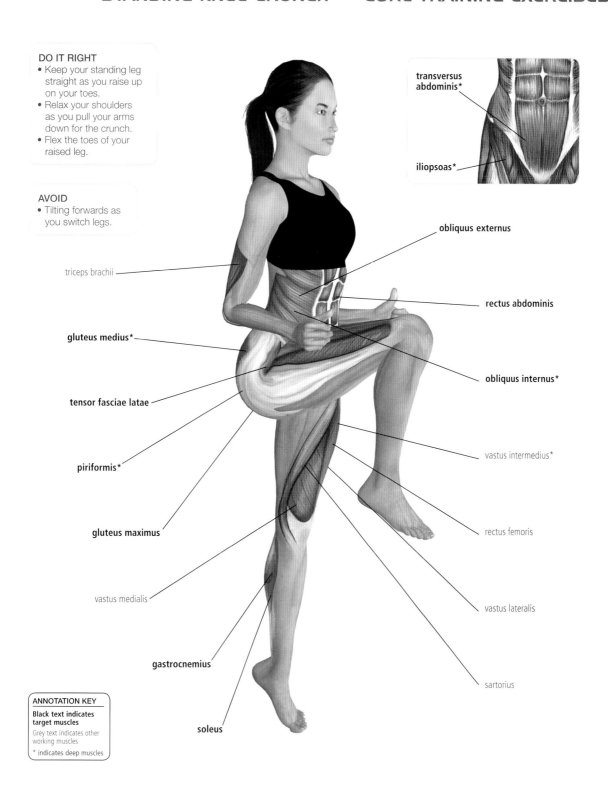

DO IT RIGHT
- Keep your standing leg straight as you raise up on your toes.
- Relax your shoulders as you pull your arms down for the crunch.
- Flex the toes of your raised leg.

AVOID
- Tilting forwards as you switch legs.

transversus abdominis*

iliopsoas*

triceps brachii

obliquus externus

rectus abdominis

gluteus medius*

obliquus internus*

tensor fasciae latae

vastus intermedius*

piriformis*

gluteus maximus

rectus femoris

vastus medialis

vastus lateralis

gastrocnemius

sartorius

soleus

ANNOTATION KEY

Black text indicates target muscles

Grey text indicates other working muscles

* indicates deep muscles

POWER SQUAT

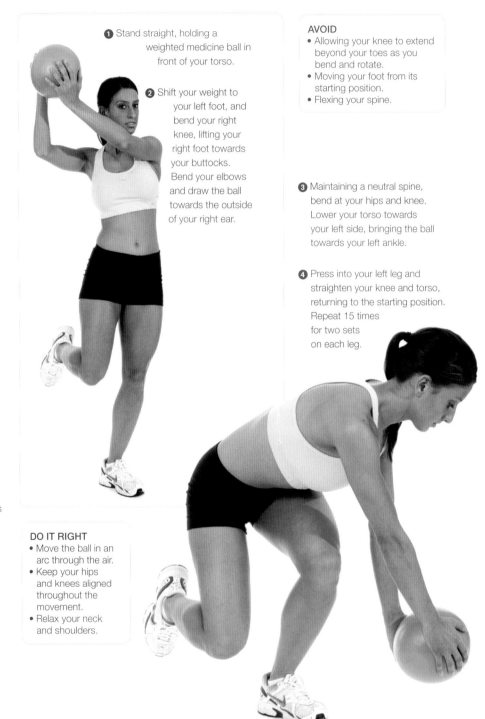

1 Stand straight, holding a weighted medicine ball in front of your torso.

2 Shift your weight to your left foot, and bend your right knee, lifting your right foot towards your buttocks. Bend your elbows and draw the ball towards the outside of your right ear.

AVOID
- Allowing your knee to extend beyond your toes as you bend and rotate.
- Moving your foot from its starting position.
- Flexing your spine.

3 Maintaining a neutral spine, bend at your hips and knee. Lower your torso towards your left side, bringing the ball towards your left ankle.

4 Press into your left leg and straighten your knee and torso, returning to the starting position. Repeat 15 times for two sets on each leg.

TARGETS
- Abdominals
- Hip flexors

LEVEL
- Advanced

BENEFITS
- Improves balance
- Stabilises pelvis, trunk and knees
- Promotes stronger movement patterns

NOT ADVISABLE IF YOU HAVE . . .
- Knee pain
- Lower-back pain
- Shoulder pain

DO IT RIGHT
- Move the ball in an arc through the air.
- Keep your hips and knees aligned throughout the movement.
- Relax your neck and shoulders.